Beyond Cohesion

PETER LANG
PROMPT

Frank A. Davis

Beyond Cohesion

Toward a Theory of Coherence

PETER LANG
Lausanne • Berlin • Bruxelles • Chennai • New York • Oxford

Library of Congress Cataloging-in-Publication Control Number: 2023002436

Bibliographic information published by the **Deutsche Nationalbibliothek.**
The German National Library lists this publication in the German
National Bibliography; detailed bibliographic data is available
on the Internet at http://dnb.d-nb.de.

Cover design by Peter Lang Group AG

ISBN 978-1-63667-103-1 (hardback)
ISBN 978-1-63667-104-8 (ebook)
ISBN 978-1-63667-105-5 (epub)
DOI 10.3726/b20665

© 2023 Peter Lang Group AG, Lausanne
Published by Peter Lang Publishing Inc., New York, USA
info@peterlang.com - www.peterlang.com

All rights reserved.
All parts of this publication are protected by copyright.
Any utilization outside the strict limits of the copyright law, without the permission of
the publisher, is forbidden and liable to prosecution.
This applies in particular to reproductions, translations, microfilming, and storage and
processing in electronic retrieval systems.

This publication has been peer reviewed.

To Chayo

Coherence is a "veritable morass, perhaps an intractable morass … one into which venturing would be ill-advised"—Edward P. J. Corbett

Contents

CHAPTER ONE: THE CONCEPT OF COHERENCE   1
   A diachronic examination of representative works demonstrates the need for identifying a comprehensive set of ways to cohere written texts for both teachers and students of rhetoric and composition. These ways form three perspectives: linguistic, cognitive, and culturally salient.
   Introduction   1
   Coherence Across the Disciplines Today   3
   A Void Within the Discipline of Rhetoric and Composition   3

CHAPTER TWO: THE LINGUISTIC PERSPECTIVE   7
   A detailed examination of three major works treating cohesion and coherence enables the linguistic elements of coherence to be identified and yields a handlist of linguistic elements of coherence. A continuum of linguistic elements of coherence follows.
   Basis for the Linguistic Perspective of Coherence   7
   The Linguistic Perspective of Coherence   10
   Halliday and Hasan   13

Gutwinski	17
Markels	21
Linguistic Elements of Coherence	27
An Explicit-Implicit Continuum	34

CHAPTER THREE THE COGNITIVE PERSPECTIVE — 37

The cognitive perspective focuses on the umbrella concepts of the given/new relationship, Gestalt psychology, and central cognitive processes. Cognitive elements, as well as linguistic elements, contribute to a coherence continuum.

Basis for the Cognitive Perspective of Coherence	37
The Cognitive Perspective of Coherence	39
Cognitive Elements of Coherence	40
Given/New Relation	40
Gestalt	42
Central Cognitive Processes	44
An Explicit-Implicit Continuum	56

CHAPTER FOUR THE CONTEXTUALLY SALIENT PERSPECTIVE — 59

Interrelationships of epistemological frames, central metaphors, sociological models, and warrants yield omnipresent and ubiquitous elements of coherence that paradoxically seldom manifest themselves in explicit forms yet remain among the most powerful of coherence elements.

Basis for the Contextually Salient Perspective	59
Central Metaphors	63
Sociological Models	70
Warrants	72
The Contextually Salient Perspective of Coherence	75
Contextually Salient Elements of Coherence	75
An Explicit-Implicit Continuum	78

CHAPTER FIVE: SYZYGY   81

*All three sets of elements—**linguistic**, cognitive, and contextually salient—interrelate in distinctive ways to achieve coherence. A visual metaphor offers a view of these elements and their interrelationships. Pedagogical implications conclude this book.*

A Visual Metaphor of Coherence   83
Points of Departure for Teachers of Rhetoric and Composition   85
Syzygy   88

Appendix   91
Works Cited   109
Index   115

CHAPTER ONE

THE CONCEPT OF COHERENCE

Introduction

Whenever we communicate through speech, coherence exists, for we humans do not communicate to not understand, but to understand and to be understood. This is not possible without coherence: coherence is the *sine qua non* for language comprehension.

Humans naturally assume that things "make sense." Thus, making sense is the unmarked condition or quality of language processing. Because coherence is so much a requisite of language processing, humans take it for granted as much as they do the solidity of the ground beneath their feet. Moreover, coherence is assumed not only of speech production, but also of written language, and indeed, of any text spoken or written. This is especially true for those of us who work in rhetoric and composition.

Documented interest in coherence dates from the classical period of rhetoric.

Aristotle, while not using the term coherence, clearly presupposes it in his *Poetics* when describing the "organic whole" as "the structural union of the parts [of the text] being such that, if any one of them is displaced or removed, the whole will be disjointed and disturbed" (35). Horace exhorts "let your work be what you will, provided only it be uniform and a whole" (68). Longinus, in "On the Sublime," tells us more: "… we see skill in invention, and due order and arrangement of matter, emerging as the hard-won result not of one thing nor of two, but of the whole texture of the composition" (43). Longinus continues

> Now, there inhere in all things by nature certain constituents which are part and parcel of their substance. It must needs be, therefore, that we shall find one source of the sublime in the systematic selection of the most important elements, and the power of forming, by their mutual combination, what may be called one body. (69)

Longinus places particular emphasis on the notion that "there inhere in all things by nature certain constituents which are part and parcel of their substance" (69). However, he does not elaborate on these "certain constituents," nor on how they "inhere in all things by nature."

According to the Oxford English Dictionary, the first recorded use of the word **coherence** in English occurred in 1604 when Robert Cawdrey published *A Table Alphabeticall of Hard English Words*, in which he listed, "cohaerence, ioning, and vniting together" (30); in 1659, Thomas Fuller used the word in *The Appeal of Injured Innocence*: "A naked sentence … disarmed of the coherence before and after it" (5); and in 1678, Thomas Hobbes made use of the word in *Decameron Physiologicum: or, Ten Dialogues of Natural Philosophy*: "… the points of Contact will be many (which make the coherence stronger)" (ix. 108).

Webster's Third New International Dictionary defines coherence as "the quality or state of cohering … systematic or methodical connectedness or interrelatedness esp. when governed by logical principles" (440).

With the word *text* meaning beyond the level of sentence and paragraph, this work uses the following definition for *coherence*: the comprehensive, systematic connection of constitutive elements of a text, with a consistent emphasis on both the totality of the text and on the interrelatedness of its constituents.

As the following pages demonstrate, *coherence* is used in a variety of disciplines, and of course, the concept of *coherence* figures most prominently in rhetoric and composition. Surprisingly, no single work within the discipline of rhetoric and composition has treated the comprehensive, systematic connection of constitutive elements of a text, with a consistent emphasis on both the totality of the text and on the interrelatedness of its constituents. *Beyond Cohesion: Toward a Theory of Coherence* does so.

Coherence Across the Disciplines Today

In a multitude of disciplines, authors use the term *coherence* in wide and varied ways. In *Metaphorical Coherence*, Aron Sjoblad uses a view of coherence to treat the relationship between body and soul in Seneca's *Epistulae*. In *The Coherence of Theism*, Richard Swinburne uses coherence as the key factor in investigating the philosophy of religion. In *Coherence, Continuity, and Cohesion: Theoretical Foundations for Document Design*, Kim Sydow Campbell offers a view of coherence based on continuity achieved primarily through Gestalt. Scholarly works in biology, chemistry, physics, and optics abound which use coherence as a principal organizing concept (G. J. Troup 1967, Davies & Spiegel 2011, Tan & Jeong 2018, and Baumgratz, Cramer, & Plenio 2014, to name a few.) In the legal field, we have works such as *Coherence: Insights from Philosophy, Jurisprudence and Artificial Intelligence*, edited by Michal Araszkiewicz and Jaromir Savelka.

A Void Within the Discipline of Rhetoric and Composition

The prior list demonstrates that the concept of coherence can figure prominently in a variety of disciplines, and we can forgive the authors of these works for assuming at face value the meaning of *coherence* and for not delving into its underlying nature; i.e., the nature of Longinus' constituent parts and how they cohere, just as we can forgive ourselves for using salt during a meal without wondering just how it is that a soft metal (sodium) and a pale green, potentially poisonous gas (chlorine) can combine to produce common salt. However, could we understand chemists who, when sprinkling salt on a salad, do not quietly marvel at the small, sparkling, octahedryl crystals because they as chemists know very well the constituent parts of salt, their properties, and their relationships? Should not we who work in rhetoric and composition also marvel at the coherence of a text because we, like chemists, do consciously know and appreciate the marvelous nature of the constituents of the text, their dynamics, and how is it that they coalesce to form multi-paragraph, multi-page, multi-chapter texts enabled through coherence, this *sine qua non* for human communication? The answer is yes, but surprisingly, it seems that we in the discipline of rhetoric and composition have too often taken the meaning of coherence for granted or relegated it to the level of sentence or paragraph and not delved into the constituent parts and the dynamics of coherence beyond the level of the paragraph, that beyond this level, a void exists concerning the *sine qua non* of language comprehension. Below, I draw on key documents to demonstrate a surprising lack of works which actually treat the underlying constituents of a text and their dynamics, especially beyond the level of paragraph.

The *CCCC Bibliography of* Composition and Rhetoric, 1987 lists "Teaching Coherence Techniques" as a subject in its index, yet of 265 entries in the indicated section, one entry deals with unity, another entry deals in part with organic form, and none deals with coherence as a topic in its own right; similarly, the bibliography lists "Coherence in Discourse" as a subject in its index, yet of 321 entries, not a single entry treats coherence as a topic in its own right, and only once does the word "coherence" even appear in the titles or abstracts of the entries (Lindemann).

The various authors of the *Harbrace College Handbook*, published in numerous editions from 1941 to the present, devote thirty-three pages to coherence: all but one of these pages focus on coherence at the sentence level.

Sanna-Kaisa Tanskanen, in *Collaborating towards Coherence: Lexical Cohesion in English Discourse* (2006), focuses on lexical cohesion, and especially on the surface features of a text.

Lester Faigley in the 2006 edition of *The Penguin Handbook* focuses on coherence at the paragraph level. Dianna Hacker and Nancy Sommers do likewise in the 2010 edition of *The Bedford Handbook*.

In the 2013 edition of the *MLA International Bibliography* under "coherence theory," only one item appears: an article in the *Journal of Ayn Rand Studies* on a theory of philosophical truth (Seddon). In the 2022 edition of the *MLA International Bibliography*, a search using "coherence theory" as key words yields forty-three entries, none of which is a book-length treatment of coherence theory for the disciplines listed above (*MLA*).

Donald Davidson, in his *American Composition and Rhetoric*, first published in 1939, devotes thirty-three pages to developing coherence in a composition, giving examples from distinguished writers which illustrate different methods of coherence; Davidson notes kinds of order— "natural," "logical," and "instinctive" (39–40) —as well as transitional devices between and within paragraphs while emphasizing concepts such as "guiding purpose" (37) and "free association" (41), but does not offer an overall view of coherence.

Edward P. J. Corbett, author of the much respected *Classical Rhetoric for the Modern Student*, supplies a wealth of detailed and systematic terms and concepts all under the rubric of classical rhetoric as demonstrated in key texts such as "Letter from Birmingham Jail," "Civil Disobedience," and "Are Women Human?," yet Corbett hardly mentions *coherence*, relegating it to the historical survey at the end of the book, linking the term to Alexander Bain, who saw *coherence* as what relates sentences to other sentences within a paragraph and to a topic (527), and Barrett Wendell, who saw *coherence* as one of a trio of key concepts, along with "unity" and "mass" (532). Perhaps we should not be surprised at this paucity, given Corbett's own view of coherence, that it is a "veritable morass" (Hall).

Linda Woodson, in her *Handbook of Modern Rhetorical Terms*, does not list coherence (nor unity nor organic form, which are traditionally associated with *belles lettres*). She does, however, list form, defining it as "The structure of the complete piece of discourse or of its identifiable parts" and likens it to dispositio in classical rhetoric (25). Such a definition, while naturally focusing on the structure of the text, fails to focus on the comprehensive, systematic interrelatedness of the text's constitutive elements.

Richard Lanham, in his *Handlist of Rhetorical Terms*, offers several related terms—composition, eutrepismus, ordo, ordinatio, synathroesmus, and taxis—but each is concerned with order, arrangement, or the putting together of words, sentences, or parts of an oration one with the other, not with their interrelatedness at the global level. Lanham writes: "Although extensively discussed in its component details, the form of the oration [the text as a whole] has not received the scholarly attention it deserves" (112).

Thus we find a surprising void regarding the *sine qua non* of language comprehension. To fill this void, I offer *Beyond Cohesion: Toward a Theory of Coherence*, a comprehensive treatment of the constitutive elements of a text beyond the level of paragraph, with a consistent emphasis on both the totality of the text and on the interrelatedness of its constituents.

Beyond Cohesion: Toward a Theory of Coherence does so through three perspectives: the linguistic, the cognitive, and the culturally salient. The linguistic perspective examines three major works that treat cohesion and coherence, identifies the linguistic elements of coherence, and offers a handlist of these elements, which, by their nature, must be explicit in a text. The cognitive perspective uses the given/new relationship, Gestalt psychology, and central cognitive processes to identify the cognitive elements of coherence, some of which may be explicit, and others, implicit. Notably, these elements are vital to both generating content and organising it in a coherent manner. The culturally salient perspective—epistemological frames, central metaphors, sociological models, and warrants—reveals a paradox, for these elements are omnipresent and ubiquitous, seldom manifest themselves in explicit forms, and yet are among the most powerful of coherence elements.

CHAPTER TWO

THE LINGUISTIC PERSPECTIVE

Basis for the Linguistic Perspective of Coherence

Several motives from a linguistic perspective drive the investigation of coherence.

One motive is the role of the tie, which is treated in some detail below, and the fact that the structural operations which enable cohesive ties are manifested in the surface language of a text very frequently and very explicitly. Unlike the cohesive ties we will encounter in the cognitive and culturally salient perspectives of coherence, whose explicit presence in the surface language of a text is often optional or not even alluded to in the text of a composition, every structural operation which enables a cohesive tie must be explicitly represented in the surface language of a text by overt markers (or by the zero marker in the case of elliptical constructions). In short, for every structural operation enabling a cohesive tie in a text, we will find a specific word or group of words in the text whose primary function is not content, but coherence.

Moreover, because markers of these structural operations, along with additional markers of coherence such as subordinators and coordinators at the clause and paragraph levels, appear the most frequently and the most explicitly in the surface language of a text, they are the most easily identified. Given the tendency in the second half of the twentieth century, at least in the United States if not in Europe, towards the analytic rather than the holistic, and the concomitant impetus to quantify data, scholars such as M. A. K. Halliday and Ruquaiya Hasan have focused on these highly frequent and explicit surface-language markers which denote the underlying, cohering structural operations of a text.

Further, this focus has been predominantly on cohesive ties at the sentence or clause level, as the ties themselves function at the sentence level, within a paragraph, across paragraphs, or throughout an entire text or composition. Such primacy of the sentence level has been disputed and called a fundamental error. Robert de Beaugrande, for example, argues that the sentence is not "the primary unit of speech production and comprehension," and cites several scholars to support his position (Ohmann; Bever, Lackner, & Kirk; Levelt).

To be sure, both speech and writing use symbols systematically, but they operate in significantly different contexts. Normal, unrehearsed speech assumes, among other things, immediate audience response in kind, and a full complement of prosodic features, as well as a full complement of gestures, all constrained by the working memory's limits of text length and complexity. Consequently, a transcript of a spoken dialog often reveals an uneven progression toward the dialog's goal, with the progression characterized by frequent fits and starts, of numerous stops and returns to the last, mutually understood point the parties of the dialog share. Such a progression is not smooth, and although produced linearly, i.e., through the speech stream, the progression is not linear.

Writing, on the other hand, subsumes all of the above characteristics of speech production as the writer engages in an inner dialog with self or with cohorts in an attempt to produce a written text, but the act of producing a composition transcends the essential and subtended characteristics of speech production because a written composition operates in a significantly different context than does speech; the context of the written composition cannot assume immediate audience response, prosodic features, or physical gestures, nor is the working memory as constrained as it is in the processing of speech; additionally, the essay or extended text, in order to be successful, must exhibit a smooth progression of thought, and it must do so within the parameters of punctuated linearity.

In order for the composition to do this, certain discrete units, with cognitive boundaries, are necessary, without which punctuated linearity gives way to undifferentiated linearity, to a gigantic run-on of notions and concepts which possesses only a faint semblance of connectivity and which fails utterly to cohere in any manner. Thus, the written text must have a basic constituent which enables its linearity to be punctuated consistently according to appropriate cognitive boundaries. This smallest constituent manifests coherence through subject-predicate relations, to use the traditional terms, or through the given-new relationship, to use more recent, cognitive terms. This "smallest" constituent is the clause.

It is both natural and logical for scholars interested in coherence from the linguistic perspective to focus predominantly on cohesive ties at the clause level as the ties themselves function within a sentence, within a paragraph, across paragraphs, or throughout an entire text or composition. In point of fact, this "smallest" constituent is incredibly complex, its study having spawned entire theoretical grammars in linguistics, such as transformational-generative grammar, and detailed pedagogical approaches in composition, such as sentence combining.

Despite this focus on the clause, we will not follow the Katz-Fodor argument that discourse consists basically of an extended and conjoined sentence. Rather, our approach to the elements of coherence will follow more inclusive arguments such as those advanced by members of the Prague School, Kenneth Pike, William Labov, Dell Hymes, and others: expressed language can be fully understood only when seen as a human action taken within a subsuming context with both explicit and implicit elements contributing to the coherence of the linguistic expression. Or, as Stephen Witte and Lester Faigley write from a more rhetorical perspective, "coherence defines those underlying semantic relations that allow a text to be understood" and "coherence conditions are governed by the writer's purpose, the audience's knowledge and expectations, and the information to be conveyed," among other things (202).

The Linguistic Perspective of Coherence

Of all the reasons which motivate scholars to investigate coherence from a linguistic perspective, perhaps the principal reason is a fascination with language, and the marvelous, but often taken-for-granted feat of learning a language. Because of the time and complexity required in learning a first language, Nature has endowed humans with an extended neoteny—the most extended of all mammals—to enable them to learn, among other things, this complicated thing called language. Amazingly, we humans do so at such a young age that most of us take language for granted and do not even remember learning it. By the age of five or so, humans have acquired a fairly complete grammar, as well as a large working vocabulary, subject to an infinite number of structural combinations in various contexts and for various purposes. Remarkably, also by this early age, these phenomenal feats of language production and comprehension have become automatic within humans, so much so that they think it as natural to use language as it is to eat and breathe. Because it is so natural and automatic, it often seems that to talk is to think, and to think is to talk, to such a degree that our inner thoughts and our "outer speech" seem one and the same, but they are not. Ideas, visualizations, and internal cognitive paradigms are not necessarily conceived or "instantiated internally" in linear fashion, yet all speech, and consequently, all writing, must comply with the physiological constraint of linearity.

Linearity accounts for much of the difficulty linguists have had in dealing with semantics and coherence. Traditionally, linguistics was limited to spoken language and to the sentence level, both of which are linear—and written language is even more constrained by linearity than is spoken language—however, semantics and coherence are not limited to linearity, and trying to treat semantics or coherence through linearity alone is like trying to define a cube using only the dimension of length without using the dimensions of height and width, or like trying to fully experience a circus while holding one's nose and plugging one's ears. This factor of linearity is the single most distinguishing characteristic between language and cognition.

Fascination with language has also led linguists to investigate the connection between language and thought. One position regarding this connection is that the dynamics of human thought are universal for all humans the world over, yet much of the linguistic aspect of human communications is not universal, but instead, particular for a specific language.

Thus, we can posit the following key tenets:

(1) underlying all languages, i.e., underlying language as *sui generis* (as a thing unto itself) is a set of cognitive universals, which in humans are "hard-wired," i. e., physiologically determined; thus, these cognitive universals are logically prior to linguistic universals (this position is articulated in chapter three);
(2) because linguistic complexity above the level of the sign develops *pari passu*, (in parallel steps) with cognitive complexity, linguistic universals have much in common with cognitive universals; thus, these *sui generis* features of language are best studied from the cognitive perspective of coherence, not the linguistic perspective;
(3) differences in languages are principally surface differences, and these differences manifest themselves in particular grammatical features of particular languages; in this work, such features are called *sui species* features and are best studied from the linguistic perspective of coherence; hence, the term **linguistic** refers to these *sui species* features.

When we distinguish cognitive universals and linguistic particulars, we see that language is a symbol system which functions in key ways to enable humans to form coherent views of that which is real in their past and present, and of that which may be possible in their future—indeed, this symbol system enables higher-order thinking itself. This symbol system, which comprises language as a thing unto itself, performs several functions, the foremost of which is reference, for it is through the symbolic function of reference that humans can "establish the temporal and logical priority of empirical reference as the original bond between external fact and conceptual thought"; all other uses of language derive from and depend on this "fundamental semantic link" (Waldron xix).

The distinction between cognitive universals and linguistic particulars also allows us to note that the systematicity of language enables humans to categorize linguistic operations peculiar to a particular language, whether the operations are primarily inflections in a language such as Russian, or primarily syntactic in a language such as English. The systematicity of English, an analytic language, allows us to identify structural operations which enable cohesive ties at various levels in a composition: between juxtaposed clauses, across non-juxtaposed clauses, between juxtaposed paragraphs, and across non-juxtaposed paragraphs. Such cohering structural operations in English include substitution, ellipsis, and co-reference.

An approach based on the distinction between cognitive universals and linguistic particulars not only reflects psychological research indicating cell specialization in the cerebral cortex, but for the teacher of language, this distinction, in combination with the notion of contextually salient features, also re-distributes the burden of communication from what has been the sole traditional carrier, the surface language of the text, to what may be called the linguistic, cognitive, and contextually salient perspectives. Significantly, this tri-partite approach also concerns itself with the feature of linearity, for the linguistic perspective is the only perspective operating under this constraint, and since it is the most explicit perspective and, indeed, the one through which the other two perspectives are related, language teachers must be particularly mindful of linearity. Consequently, they must also pay especial attention to directionality of reference—anaphoric, cataphoric, or exophoric, for example—and how it relates to the nucleus of natural-language logic, a nucleus consisting of reference and logical identity; these concepts are discussed in the context of Halliday and Hasan's work on cohesion.

What follows is a survey of three major works which treat elements of coherence from three perspectives: from the linguistic perspective, M. A. K. Halliday and Ruquaiya Hasan's *Cohesion in English*, from the perspective of *belles lettres*, Waldemar Gutwinski's *Cohesion in Literary Texts*, and from the compositionist's perspective, Robin Markels' *A New Perspective in Cohesion in Expository Paragraphs*. The survey ends with the identification of elements of coherence from the linguistic perspective and their placement along an explicit-implicit continuum.

Halliday and Hasan

Halliday and Hasan's *Cohesion in English* is the single most cited work on the topic of cohesion. Scholars such as Waldemar Gutwinski even regard Halliday and Hasan's treatment of cohesion as the ultimate position on textual cohesion, but this position may well be like that of such linguists as Leonard Bloomfield, Charles Fries, and other structuralists who believed the study of language had reached its zenith in the late 1950s when methods of linguistic analysis enabled the "complete description of all human languages." Studies in neuro-, psycho-, and sociolinguistics now indicate the fallacy of this position. Nonetheless, Halliday and Hasan's treatment of cohesion in English merits attention for it deals intricately with the most explicit and most frequently used elements of coherence.

Halliday and Hasan's method of textual analysis, is, in their words, a "way to offer an insight into what it is that makes a text a text" (328), and to do so they place cohesion within a "description of English," with the sentence as the "highest structural unit in their grammar" (28). Linguistic structures are limited to four "ranks": clause, verbal group, nominal group, and adverbial group. Despite these limits, however, Halliday and Hasan investigate the "linguistic means whereby a text is enabled to function as a single meaningful unit" (29–30). Further, a "text," i.e., a sentence, exhibits "texture" when it "functions as a unity with respect to its environments" (2). According to Halliday and Hasan, texture is achieved through the mutually complementary relationship of "register" and "cohesion" (23). Here, we see Halliday and Hasan tending toward coherence via extra-textual features with the mention of register, but they pull back. Indeed, as Patricia Carrell in "Cohesion is Not Coherence" tells us, according to Halliday and Hasan, "cohesion is not a matter of content or textual meaning" (481).

Halliday and Hasan posit five cohesive, "non-structural components of the semantic system" of English: reference, substitution, ellipsis, conjunction, and lexical cohesion (29). Halliday and Hasan argue that these components figure centrally in the cohesion of a text.

In treating the following passage from *Alice in Wonderland*, Halliday and Hasan identify the components of reference, substitution, ellipsis, conjunction, and lexical cohesion as they function to cohere the passage:

> [1:5a] The Cat only grinned when it saw Alice.
>   "Come, it's pleased so far," thought Alice, and she went on. "Would you tell me, please, which way I ought to go from here?"
>   "That depends a good deal on where you want to get to," said the Cat.
>   "I don't much care where—" said Alice.
>   "Then it doesn't matter which way you go," said the Cat.
>   "—so long as I get *somewhere*" Alice added as an explanation. "Oh, you're sure to do that," said the Cat, "if you only walk long enough."
>
> (in Halliday & Hasan 30)

Working from the last lines to the first, Halliday and Hasan argue that "do that" SUBSTITUTES for "get *somewhere*," which is tied through LEXICAL COHESION to "where you want to get to," which is related also through LEXICAL COHESION to "which way I ought to go." "Oh" serves as a CONJUNCTION for "—so long as I get somewhere" and "you're sure to do that," and "then" also serves as a CONJUNCTION as it coheres "I don't much care where—" to "… it doesn't matter which way you go." In Alice's second utterance, ELLIPSIS coheres "where" with the Cat's second utterance "… where you want to get to," and LEXICAL COHESION ties Alice's "care" with the Cat's "want." REFERENCE ties "that" in the Cat's first utterance to Alice's question "… which way I ought to go," and, again, REFERENCE ties "it" of Alice's interior monologue to "The Cat" in the first line of the passage. Throughout the passage, from its beginning to its end, REPETITION ties "Alice" and "the Cat" into a "cohesive chain" (30).

If, in the illustration on the following page, *italics*, **bold**, ***bold italics***, and underlining indicate the words in the passage which cohere through ties and ALL-CAPITALS denote the words which actually tie (which are conjunctions, at least in this passage). If lines of coherence are drawn connecting the elements of each cohesive tie, the manner in which this passage is bound together begins to take shape. The elements of coherence in this or any passage effect lines of coherence which exert a binding and unifying force not only between themselves, but also on much of the content within them or near the lines of coherence.

[1:5b] **The Cat** only grinned when **it** saw *Alice*. "Come, **it**'s pleased so far," thought *Alice*, and *she* went on. "Would **you** tell *me*, please, ***which way** I* ought to go from here?"
"***That*** depends a good deal on ***where you*** want to get to," said **the Cat**.
"*I* don't much care ***where***" said *Alice*. "THEN ***it*** doesn't matter ***which way you*** go," said **the Cat**.
"--so long as *I* get somewhere" *Alice* added as an explanation.
"OH, *you*'re sure to do that," said **the Cat**, if *you* only walk long enough."

Thus Halliday and Hasan's approach begins to shed light on the linguistic aspects of coherence, but the analysis of the sample passage also raises questions. For example, pronouns substitute for Alice or the Cat ten times, and **it** substitutes once for an entire clause ("I don't much care where [I get to].") Are these pronouns, which serve as substitutes for **Alice** or **the Cat**, and which Halliday and Hasan do not note, a part of the "cohesive chain" represented by the repetition of **Alice** or **the Cat**?

We might also observe that repetition is not included among Halliday and Hasan's five elements of cohesion, yet they explicitly use this term as it serves a consistent cohesive function throughout the passage. Interestingly, of Halliday and Hasan's five sub-categories of cohesion, (or six, if one counts repetition), only one—conjunction—has words in the text which actually tie, i.e., THEN and OH, while the remaining sub-categories of cohesion do not act as ties, but instead enable coherence by representing a cohesive tie brought about by a structural operation, i.e., substitution, ellipsis, and co-reference, or by a semantic relation, i.e., lexical cohesion, and repetition. (Because I reduce a significant portion of Halliday and Hasan's *Cohesion in English* to a small number of elements which contribute fundamentally to the theory of coherence, and because I do not want to seem peremptory in this reduction, I offer in the appendix a multi-paged argument concerning these conclusions for those who wish to work through the details.)

In sum, Halliday and Hasan make a valuable contribution to the linguistic perspective of coherence through their delineation and examination of such cohesive operations as the tie, co-reference, substitution, ellipsis, conjunction, and lexical cohesion. Moreover, *Cohesion in English* offers valuable insight into how structural operations, especially those involving substitution of pro-forms or the zero element, comprise the lion's share of the cohesive elements in the linguistic perspective of coherence.

However, as the argument in the appendix demonstrates, co-reference and ellipsis are forms of substitution (see A10 in the appendix), and substitution is structural in nature (A10, A12, and A13), being achieved through structural operations in English as shown by transformational-generative grammar. These structural operations enable cohesive ties which, with few exceptions, are explicitly represented in the surface language of a text by overt markers as catalogued below in this chapter and which are essential for logical identity, which, along with symbolic reference, constitutes the nucleus of natural language logic. This nucleus is encompassed by the linguistic, cognitive, and contextually salient perspectives as the visual metaphor in chapter five illustrates.

Thus, although Halliday and Hasan nominally reject any extratextual considerations of coherence, their focus on *sui species* (species specific) features of a text's surface language, viz., repetition (of co-referents), anaphora and cataphora (relating to pro-forms and directionality of reference), and ellipsis (substitution of the zero element), constitute the basic ties and thus are fundamental to this investigation of the linguistic perspective of coherence. Yet, we need to add that as fundamental as they are, "ties are not, by themselves, sufficient to create coherent text" (Bamberg 418) as we shall see in chapters three and four of this work.

Gutwinski

Waldemar Gutwinski's *Cohesion in Literary Texts*, published in the same year as Halliday and Hasan's *Cohesion in English* and drawing from Halliday and Hasan's earlier publications (Halliday and Hasan 1962, 1964, 1972; Hasan 1964, 1967, 1968), posits a theoretical framework quite similar to that of Halliday and Hasan in terms of cohesive elements. As the title indicates, Gutwinski focuses on works in *belles lettres*, and he analyzes passages by Ernest Hemingway and Henry James, whereas Halliday and Hasan offer a more purely linguistic approach using mainly dialog and narrative.

We should note at the outset that although Gutwinski touches on research concerning coherence, he believes coherence to be unanalyzable in the linguistic sense because it deals with phenomena which "cannot be treated on a single level of analysis and some of which are not open to linguistic analysis at all" (26). These latter "phenomena" are things such as "gaps in thought," which Gutwinski illustrates with a brief passage from a first-year composition text, *Writing with a Purpose*, in which the author, James McCrimmon, advises student writers to avoid "gaps in thought" if they wish to write a coherent paragraph. Thus, Gutwinski tells us, the term **coherence** is "carefully avoided" in his work (27).

Gutwinski states that none of the "several competing theories of language organization [the extended standard theory of generative transformational grammar, generative semantics, applicational-generative, tagmemic, systemic, and stratificational grammar] …" has "developed a semology or fully-worked out tactics for its upper stratum (lexical hierarchy or lexis)" which "must be seen as an inadequacy if any explicitness is attempted" (23). This view notwithstanding, Gutwinski uses stratificational theory as his theoretical base because "it recognizes and develops several strata, one of which is semology" (25); this semology is defined as a system "behind" grammar that consists of

> meaning contrasts and patterns of sense organization … [which are] still very poorly understood. Yet we suspect that the relationship of semology to grammar is much the same as that of grammar to phonology. (Gleason qtd. in Gutwinski 1976, 39)

Gutwinski relates that most of the linguistic phenomena in his approach belong to the "grammatic stratum" (*sic*) of stratificational grammar (25). He thus proceeds to examine "the cohesive relations obtaining between clauses and sentences in some selected literary prose texts," that is, passages from James and Hemingway (26).

Several "cohesive categories" are offered by Gutwinski (54), the foremost of which is "the method of order" of sentences (55). He states:

> The order in which clauses and sentences follow in a text is, then, a cohesive factor which is always present in the text and which in combination with other cohesive factors—and sometimes even alone—indicates what kind of cohesive relations obtain among the sentence and clauses it [order] will underlie implicitly ... involving all other cohesive factors studied here. (Gutwinski 56)

Unfortunately, Gutwinski develops nothing further *vis-a-vis* order and these "implicit correlations." Instead, he focuses on much the same sort of cohesive relations that Halliday and Hasan do. Gutwinski divides cohesive features into two categories, grammatical and lexical. The grammatical category consists of anaphora/cataphora, coordination/subordination, and enation/agnation; the lexical category consists of repetition, occurrence of a synonym or item "formed on same root," and occurrence of an "item from same lexical set (co-occurrence group)" (57).

Gutwinski, drawing from Gleason, enlarges the "phoric" category to include not only anaphora and cataphora, but also homophora (reference to general or cultural knowledge, e.g., "the army," "the queen," "the Superbowl"), exophora (reference to "a situation outside of language," e.g., using a gesture to supplement our communication), and paraphora (reference to something in another text, e.g., a line from Shakespeare) (66–68); however, Gutwinski's approach does not admit any reference other than anaphora or cataphora, presumably for the same reasons he avoids all use of the word **coherence**: such aspects, in his approach, are non-linguistic. Although Gutwinski admits only anaphora and cataphora for his approach to cohesion, we can relate all five kinds of "phoric" reference to the notion of linearity, the significant constraint under which the linguistic perspective must operate, but which the cognitive and contextually salient perspectives are free of.

Both Gutwinski and Halliday and Hasan give considerable attention to anaphora and cataphora, with Gutwinski arguing (60–61) that anaphora has traditionally received the most attention of all cohesive features, with that attention initially focused within clauses (Bloomfield 1933), but that later scholars have broadened the scope to include interclausal cohesion (Gleason; Halliday & Hasan; Quirk, Greenbaum, Leech, & Svartvik). We might add that both anaphora and cataphora adhere to the constraint of linearity and are distinguished one from the other primarily in terms of directionality. Paraphora, too, is constrained by linearity, but it is the linearity of another text, and thus it is disallowed *per* Gutwinski's criteria. We might argue that paraphora is a type of homophora. We can also note that much of these two fundamental kinds of reference is not constrained by linearity, and that they are within the bounds of the contextually salient perspective of coherence.

Again drawing from Gleason, Gutwinski illustrates enation and agnation as grammatical features. Enation, a form of grammatical parallelism, is illustrated by the following nursery rhyme:

> [2:71] This little pig went to market This little pig stayed home. This little pig had roast beef.
> This little pig had none (76).

Agnation is "used for relations that are opposite and complementary to enation" (78). The following sentences illustrate agnation:

> [2:72] There was nothing left for her but to sell the old family house. This she couldn't do.

This she couldn't do is an agnate structure which serves to cohere the two sentences by reversing the SVO word order of **sell the old house**. However, we might also argue that **This**, in conjunction with **do**, are substitutes for **sell the old family house**, and that **This** has been fronted through a structural operation akin to the do-fronting transformation in transformational-generative grammar, and that the variation in word order is not as much for purposes of cohesion as for stylistic emphasis. One other example of agnation is the following:

[2:73] James wrote this book.
This book was written by James. (78)

Here we have an example of the active-passive transformation. The reason for the alternation between structures lies not so much in efforts to cohere a text via structural operations as in the given/new relationship, which, it will be argued in chapter three of this book, is a fundamental part of the cognitive perspective.

Gramatical and Lexical Ties

In sum, Gutwinski offers two main categories, the grammatical and the lexical, whose elements serve as overt markers of cohesive ties and which are explicitly represented in the surface language of a text. The grammatical category consists of anaphora/cataphora, coordination/subordination, and enation/agnation: the lexical category consists of repetition, occurrence of synonyms, and co-occurrence of items from the same lexical group. Yet, as was argued earlier, coordination and subordination might be better treated from the cognitive perspective because of their close relationship to central cognitive processes. Enation, to the extent it is cohesive rather than stylistic, might be better treated from the contextually salient perspective since parallelism is one of several cultural thought patterns that humans use to structure their thought and text (Kaplan). As stated earlier, agnation might be better treated from the cognitive perspective due to its representing the given/new relationship. Those cohesive ties represented by synonyms and items from the same lexical group might best be treated as part of natural or synthetic semantic domains, with the former viewed from the cognitive perspective and the latter from the contextually salient perspective. This leaves repetition, anaphora, and cataphora; the latter two result from structural operations as demonstrated by transformational generative grammar, and are forms of substitution differing primarily in directionality. Although Halliday and Hasan also mentioned repetition as a cohesive operation, they did not elaborate on it or assign it to a cohesive category other than to state that it is a type of reiteration (Halliday & Hasan 278).

Halliday & Hasan, Gutwinski: Repetition, Anaphora, Cataphora, Ellipsis Are the Basic Ties

The review of Gutwinski and Halliday and Hasan indicates that the basic cohesive categories in the linguistic perspective continue to emanate from the fundamental structural operation of substitution: for Halliday and Hasan, the cohesive categories are co-reference, ellipsis, and substitution, with co-reference and ellipsis being types of substitution, and for Gutwinski, the cohesive categories are anaphora, cataphora, and repetition, with anaphora and cataphora kinds of co-reference, and therefore examples of substitution.

In addition to reinforcing the primacy of substitution as a cohesive tie in the linguistic perspective, Gutwinski expands the notion of reference by drawing on Gleason's work on "phoric" reference. Gutwinski not only treats anaphoric and cataphoric reference in relation to cohesion, but he also treats homophoric, paraphoric, and exophoric reference. Although he does not admit the three as cohesive, our approach to coherence, consisting of not only the linguistic perspective, but also the cognitive and contextually salient perspectives, will admit these latter three types of reference, and hence, they will be related to in the respective chapters of this book. Moreover, Gutwinski's treatment of the various kinds of "phoric" reference enables us to relate each to the notion of linearity, which, as was noted earlier, is a significant constraint for the linguistic perspective, but not for the cognitive nor the contextually salient perspectives.

Markels

Markels' work, *A New Perspective on Cohesion in Expository Paragraphs*, offers interesting points of commonality and dissimilarity with respect to the works of Gutwinski and of Halliday and Hasan. Where Gutwinski focuses on works of *belles lettres* and Halliday and Hasan focus mainly on dialog and narrative, Markels focuses on expository writing; where Gutwinski is oriented toward the text as a whole and Halliday and

Hasan are oriented towards texts of various lengths exhibiting various degrees of closure, Markels is oriented toward paragraphs. In addition, Markels does not offer an overall framework for analyzing the elements of coherence as do Gutwinski and Halliday and Hasan. In these ways, Markels' treatment of the linguistic aspect of differs markedly from those of Gutwinski and Halliday and Hasan. These significant differences notwithstanding, Markels finds common ground with both Gutwinski and Halliday and Hasan in two key areas: (1) the essential roles of substitution, ellipsis, and [co-]reference in cohering a text; and, (2) the essential and subsuming role of repetition in cohering a text.

Recurrence (repetition) Chains

Central to Markels' approach is the notion of recurrence; indeed, she argues that "Where a recurrence chain exists, there is cohesion; without a chain, [there is] no cohesion" (14). Although she does not cite Harris, it would seem that Markels' notion of a recurrence chain is quite similar to Harris' "equivalence chain" (6–29); however, Harris explores the use of the equivalence chain through various grammatical structures and lexical domains, while Markels by-and-large restricts her examination of "recurrence chains" to the three structural operations of substitution, ellipsis, and co-reference, all three of which she states are "forms of partial repetition" (17). We should note, though, that although for Markels the notion of recurrence is central to her approach, her view of recurrence goes beyond the notion that it is simply repetition, whether it is manifested through the structural operations of substitution, ellipsis, or co-reference, or whether it is "simply" the repeated use of the same word. For Markels, this expanded notion of recurrence comprises the principal property of linguistic cohesion. Markels illustrates this centrality by using the following two examples:

> [2:74] The opossum has survived in definitely hostile surroundings for seventy million years. The opossum is small; it can easily find a little food, while big animals starve. The individual opossum is not very delicate; it can stand severe punishment. It "plays 'possum" when it gets into trouble. It can go without food for a long time. Many different things are food to an opossum. Traits of the opossum have a high

survival value. The opossum is a survivor from the Age of Reptiles. (qtd. in Gorrell & Laird 125)

[2:75] The reasons our opossum has survived in definitely hostile surroundings for 70 million years are evident. One is his small size: small animals always find hiding places; they always find a little food, where the big ones starve. Another of its assets was its astounding fecundity; if local catastrophes left only a few survivors, it did not take long to reestablish a thriving population. Also the individual opossum is not exactly delicate: it can stand severe punishment—during which it "plays 'possum" and then scampers away—and it can go without food for a considerable time. Finally, a great many things are "food" to an opossum. Each of these traits has a high survival value, and their combination has presented the United States with a survivor from the Age of Reptiles. (qtd. in Gorrell & Laird 126)

In the first opossum text, the recurrence chain is established through simple repetition of the word **opossum**; in the second opossum text (organized as an argument), the recurrence chain is established not only by the word **opossum**, but also through the structural operations of substitution, ellipsis, and co-reference, and such structural operations, Markels argues, function in two important ways: (1) they "maintain an unbroken chain of recurrences and thereby establish some degree of cohesion through unity"; and (2) they "subordinate information already known or recoverable by reducing the autonomy of sentences containing that information and forcing the reader back to preceding sentences for the antecedents or other substitutions" (17).

To bolster her argument that repetition is central to cohesion, Markels points out that in various psycholinguistic studies concerned with thematization (Perfetti & Goldman; Kintsch; Bransford & Franks; and Crothers), the "shared constant" was repetition, except in the work of Crothers, who concedes that lack of repetition "probably explains his negative results" (38). This, Markels states, confirms her hypothesis that "cohesion consists primarily of unity, the presence of a repeated term" (38).

Single-term and Multiple-chain Paragraphs

To demonstrate her approach, Markels analyzes two kinds of paragraphs, single-term and multiple-chain. Here we examine her analysis of a single-term paragraph, i.e., a paragraph whose cohesion is established through one recurrence chain, as opposed to a multiple-chain paragraph which may have a dominant recurrence chain and subordinate recurrence chains.

Cohesion in the single-term paragraph occurs when "a term achieves semantic dominance through repetition or equivalence" and "appears consistently in the subject or dominant noun phrase position" (45), as in the following "basic" paragraph

> [2:76] The Char-Bar is a bar on High Street. The Char-Bar swings. It permits dancing. The bar specializes in foreign beers. The Char-Bar attracts weirdos. It seats 198 people.

as opposed to the set of sentences below, which possesses a semantically dominant term, but not one that appears consistently in the subject or dominant noun phrase position:

> [2:77] Alfred likes peaches. Oregon doesn't grow peaches. Peaches contain nitrogen. We have a peach tree in our backyard. No one throws rotten peaches at politicians or ball players. Cut five peaches and sprinkle with sugar. Do you think peach melba would be a good dessert?

Referring to example [2:77], Markels states that "once the repeated term 'peaches' appears in the predicate position, it forfeits the inherently limiting power of the subject position and is itself 'subjected' to at least five other topics: Alfred, Oregon, we, no one, you." Markels continues by observing that "cohesion requires the meshing of both semantic and syntactic information and, at least for some paragraphs ... can be defined operationally" (44).

Semantics vs. Syntax

At this juncture, it might be good to note that structure, as opposed to syntax alone, occupies a prominent role in this work's three-pronged approach to coherence, and that structure in this work is confined neither to syntax nor to the linguistic perspective. Indeed, it is argued in chapters three and four that structure forms an essential aspect of both the cognitive and contextually salient perspectives of. Thus, it can be pointed out that in example [2:77], more than simply placing the word **peach** in the subject position of each sentence would be required to cohere the collection of sentences into a paragraph, as the "re-structuring" below indicates:

> [2:78] Peaches are a favorite of Alfred's. Peaches don't grow in Oregon. A peach tree grows in our backyard. Peaches are not thrown at politicians or ball players. Five peaches are cut and sprinkled with sugar. Peach melba would be a good dessert, don't you think?

Although the "Char-Bar" paragraph [2:76] will never win a prize for style, it at least is coherent; as for paragraph [2:78], not even moving the word **peach** to the subject position can salvage this poor collection of sentences.

Markels' assertion to the contrary, it would seem that a cohesive paragraph subtends more than a meshing of semantics and syntax; it is a meshing of more than these two important elements, and chapters three and four will illuminate, at least in part, other elements which serve to provide a coherent text. Perhaps part of the problem in Markels' semantics-syntax argument lies in two of her premises.

> The first premise is that English is "position dependent on syntactic information" (45).

Markels does not elaborate on what she means by syntactic information, and of course, English is primarily an SVO language. However, as the wealth of sentence variety due to variation in word order illustrates, English is *not* position dependent for syntactic information, as examples [2:77] and [2:78] show.

The second premise is that a transformational analysis can illustrate the

> semantic-syntax relationship by using the TG concept of dominant sentence node when a collection of sentences employs ellipsis in lieu of term repetition. This premise overlooks the fundamental non-semantic nature of TG sentence trees. As Chomsky and others have repeatedly shown, TG grammar was concerned with syntax, not semantics. Moreover, a non-sensical sentence tree employing elliptical constructions is easily

generated because transformational grammar deals with sentence structure, not sentence sense.

It is interesting to note that while Markels stresses that her approach is "[h]eavily grounded in syntactic analysis" (86) and places the burden of cohesion on "the meshing of both semantic and syntactic information" (44), thus confining the role of structure to syntactic structure, she seems to anticipate cognitive and contextually salient elements of coherence, for she states that "[o]nly the concept of an a priori frame" composed of a world view between the communicants can "explain language use" (33), citing research which supports this view (Minsky 1975; Schank & Abelson 1974; Rommetveit 1974). Such a reference to *a priori* frames suggests the kind of "hard-wired" central cognitive processes to be explored in chapter three of this work, and Markels' mention of world views, and concomitantly, extra-textual elements, suggests the concepts of central metaphors and epistemological frames which are treated in chapter four of this work. Likewise, Markels seems to anticipate contextually salient elements of coherence when she reflects on the role subjective interpretation plays whenever a person engages with a text. She quotes Stephen Tyler in his *The Said and the Unsaid: Mind, Meaning, and Culture*: the "objective and universal character ... [of a text and its textuality] ... can be realized only through the subjectivity of some reader, thus the burden of interpretation" (378).

In sum, Markels does not offer an overall framework which subsumes categories and elements of cohesion as do the authors of the other two major works on cohesion, Gutwinski and Halliday and Hasan; in addition, Markels' focus is primarily on paragraphs, not on texts comprised of paragraphs. We might also disagree with her premises concerning the role of syntax *vis-a-vis* cohesion in paragraphs. Finally, Markels does not explore the nature and various manifestations of "phoric" reference as do Gutwinski and Halliday and Hasan. However, we may observe that she, unlike Gutwinksi and Halliday and Hasan, seems to allow for non-linguistic, i.e., non-textual, elements in the coherence of a text.

In Conclusion of the Survey of Halliday and Hasan, Gutwinski, and Markels

Significantly, Markels reiterates the aspects of cohesion that both Gutwinski and Halliday and Hasan find central to coherence: repetition, anaphora, cataphora, and ellipsis.

Linguistic Elements of Coherence

As noted earlier, the linguistic perspective deals with those elements manifested the most frequently and often the most explicitly in a text; such elements are manifested through and by a text's own language in words meant to be understood at the literal level. As a review of *Cohesion in English, Cohesion in Literary Texts,* and *A New Perspective on Cohesion in Expository Paragraphs* indicates, these elements are indeed text-bound, and therefore significantly constrained by linearity, hence the emphases on repetition, anaphora, cataphora, and ellipsis by Halliday and Hasan, Gutwinski, and Markels. Our review of the above-mentioned works also reveals that an additional constraint operates in the linguistic perspective: the constraint of co-reference. Thus, we can make the generalization that linguistic elements of coherence are meant to be understood at the literal level of language and are constrained by the properties of linearity and co-reference.

When we determine to form a cohesive tie, whether immediate, mediated, or remote, we must choose whether the tie will be explicit or have a significant degree of implicitness.

If we choose an explicit tie, three options exist: repetition of the referent, an anaphoric pro-form co-referential with the referent, or a cataphoric pro-form co-referential with the referent. If we choose a tie with a significant degree of implicitness, only one option exists: ellipsis, which, though almost always anaphoric, is largely implicit in nature because of its "zero component."

Thus, linguistic elements of coherence are represented by four categories: repetition, ellipsis, anaphora, and cataphora. Of these four categories, the latter three appear in the surface structure of a text through structural operations of the sort illustrated by transformational-generative grammar. The remaining category, repetition, appears via duplication of the referent or substitution of an equivalent term. The elements of repetition, i.e., the words used to enable repetition, constitute an open set since it consists of repetition of the referent or substitution of an equivalent term, and the referent may be represented by any number of constructions or word classes. The elements of ellipsis also constitute an open set since its surface manifestations may be represented by any number of constructions and word classes. The elements of anaphora and the elements of cataphora constitute closed sets—those of pro-forms.

The Four Categories of the Linguistic Elements of Coherence

Repetition (open set) duplication of the referent itself or substitution of an equivalent term

Ellipsis (open set)
(substitution by the zero element of a portion of a parallel and recoverable form)

Anaphora (closed set) above
The source for the **above** figures for the deficit is the Congressional Office of the Budget.

aforementioned

The **aforementioned** plat is erroneous in both scale and orientation.

be

We will be visiting Africa in 1999 for the entire summer, and Mark and Carol also will **be**.

be it

Paco Sinmiedo will find his name in *The Guinness Book of Records*, **be it** next year or the following one.

be so

>Mother seems always to be tired, irritable, and sleepy. I don't want her to **be so**.

be that
>She proposes to continue college after the birth of her twins, **be that** feasible or not.

do
>Democrats want the economy to improve; Republicans and independents **do**, too.

do it
>Jonathan doesn't care how long it takes him to secure a good position. He just wants to **do it**.

do so
>You want me to examine the tires, the carburetor, and the brakes, and I will **do so**, but please let me eat lunch first.

do that
>The police officer asked me to get into his cruiser, but I refused to **do that**.

do the same
>Martin Luther King, Jr. achieved a measure of civil rights success, and it became clear that Malcom X wanted to **do the same**.

he
>John is a solid fellow; **he** is always honest and considerate.

her
>Sally dances wonderfully; I could have danced all night with **her**.

here
>The Versailles Treaty is much too severe, and **here** the Allied Powers err tragically.

hers

> Let me see Cecilia's paintings; **hers** are always worth buying.

him

> I liked George very much, but I could never understand **him**.

his

> I want to see Jeff's notes because **his** are easier to read.

identical

> The first superchip was manufactured in Silicon Valley, but an **identical** one was soon manufactured in Hamburg.

it

> Approving the budget will be difficult, but **it** is vital.

its

> Examine the dog's left-rear paw; **its** webbing has been torn.

likewise

> Lafayette was given honorary citizenship, and **likewise**, Churchill.

not

> He says that to juggle the accounts to achieve his promotion is the surest and quickest way to advance in the firm, but it is **not**.

one

> Both students studied hard, but only **one** passed the exam.

ones

> Yes, I know there are all sorts of onions, but only the **ones** from Valdalia are sweet enough to eat like an apple.

same

> Ellen wrote her first novel at age twenty-six, and I did the **same**.

she

> My first Spanish teacher will always by my favorite, for **she** is the one I married.

so

> Joanna hopes to be home for Christmas. I hope **so**, too.

so + adjective/adverb

> The theater was absolutely crowded. I did not expect **so many** people at this performance.

such + adjective + noun phrase

> I love purple. It is **such a royal color**.

that

> As the young woman accepted the bouquet of flowers, she smiled and said "**That** was a gracious gesture on your part."

that + adjective/adverb

> Rueckert broke the four-minute mark! I had no idea he ran **that fast**!

the

> A young man stood alone at the highest point of the bridge. **The** young man was Stephen Daedelus.

the aforesaid

> The aforesaid is not the man we are after.

the earlier

> The cinema has two matinees on Sundays. **The earlier** has seats for only one dollar.

the first (second, third, ...)

> **The first** was the best.

the foregoing

> No matter how you argue, **the foregoing** will need to be notarized.

the former/the latter

> Sonny Liston and Muhammad Ali were two heavyweight champions of the world.
> **The former** was an ex-con, and **the latter** was an extra-good con.

the last

> **The last** actually scored better because of the softened playing field.

the preceding

> **The preceding** was unnecessary propaganda. Everyone is already convinced.

the said

> **The said** will be arraigned on Saturday at noon.

their

> Tolstoy and Dostoevsky have long been dead, but **their** influence continues.

theirs

> I have eaten my hamburger, but Sam and Dave have not; **theirs** is on the stove.

them

> Your sister and your brother will be here for only two more weeks. We must do our best to entertain **them**.

then

> I opened the door casually; it was **then** that I realized the room was decorated and all my friends were waiting for me.

there

> The does frolicked in the meadow, and **there** the youth photographed them.

these

>The student had split an infinitive and ended a sentence with a preposition. The infuriated teacher shouted **"These** are the kinds of errors which I will not tolerate!"

they

>Mssrs. Reagan and Bush were both traditional Republicans in that **they** relied heavily on defense spending.

this

>The hardliners underestimated Mr. Gorbachev, and **this** was a mistake.

those

>"Give me Socrates, Plato, and Zorba! **Those** are the Greeks I am most interested in!".

which

>I ran seven miles the day I decided to begin my diet, **which** was not the prudent thing to do.

Cataphora (closed set)

as follows

>The criteria are **as follows**: six foot minimum height, six foot minimum depth, and four foot minimum width.

below

>**Below**, you will find the necessary instructions for complete assembly of the rocking horse.

here

>**Here** is where you are wrong. Inflation will not soar out of control as long as the Federal Reserve maintains tight control of the money supply.

it

>**It** is wonderful to be independent.

the following

> The successful definition must include **the following**: the placing of the term within a class; the distinguishing of the term from other items in the class; an example illustrating the term.

these

> **These** are the latest photographs of Mars.

this

> **This** is what will happen next. The lioness will actually purr her way out of the fix she is in!

thus

> "It is **thus**," intoned the piano teacher, after which his long, slender fingers nimbly scaled the notes.

thusly

> The Prussian drill instructor yelled "You will do **thusly**!" Then, he demonstrated an about-face, followed by the clicking of his heels.

An Explicit-Implicit Continuum

As noted in the overview of the linguistic perspective, a language is a marvelously complex and prolific system of symbols. This symbol system is so rich and so variegated that it complements the richness and variegation of the human mind in a *pari passu* relationship, thus enabling humans to achieve levels of thought much higher than the level of sign.

The richness and variegation of this symbol system is evident when we consider that in English 26 letters form approximately 500,000 words, and of these 500,000 words, we can form an infinite number of sentences. It is this unlimited combinatorial nature that we must wrestle with and express ourselves through as we attempt to make sense of our surroundings and life. Fortunately, this burgeoning infinity of language is made manageable through the logic of natural language. At the very nucleus of this logic are the semantically primal qualities of symbolic reference and logical identity. Symbolic reference enables the symbol to re-present for the language user the referent, and, as Waldron demonstrates, is not a mundane affair, but one having significant cognitive implications which chapter three will treat within the rubric of the cognitive elements of coherence.

Symbolic reference is distinguished by polysemy, yet this very characteristic, which elevates sign to symbol, thereby affording to it greater utility, also affords to it greater potential for ambiguity or confusion. This liability is offset, however, by the second nuclear quality of natural language logic, logical identity, for logical identity not only helps us winnow the several meanings a term may have, but it also enables us to view the item with a consistent meaning throughout a text, and it is here that the significance of the linguistic elements of coherence becomes evident.

If we compare the very small number of anaphoric and cataphoric elements to the half million-plus words available in the English language, and, as will be done in chapters three and four, if we compare the essentially explicit nature of these linguistic elements to the relatively implicit nature of the cognitive and contextually salient elements of, we may rightly be intrigued by their prominence in the overall schema of coherence: upon analysis, we find that their small number is offset by their high frequency of usage. Further, we find that their word class, their relatively small number and high frequency, and their mandatory explicitness enable logical identity.

If we hold that symbolic reference is rooted in, but not restricted to, empirical experience, if we follow Wolfgang Dressler and others who posit that semantic deep structure consists solely of noun phrases, and further, that the overwhelming use of symbolic reference is not empirical reference, i.e., referring exclusively to the empirical here-and-now, but instead, that most language use is modal reference, i.e., referring to all situations and circumstances not in the empirical here-and-now (Waldron), we can see that the properties of word class, of relatively small number and high frequency, and of mandatory explicitness enable the linguistic elements of coherence to serve an essential role in the cohering of discourse.

The dominant word class for the linguistic elements of coherence is that of pro-forms or their derivatives, even in elliptical constructions (e.g., the possessive pronouns **his** and **hers**). These pro-forms are either full or truncated noun phrases and represent surface manifestations quite similar to the corresponding noun phrase in semantic deep structure. The small number and high frequency of the linguistic elements of coherence ease memory load, increase clarity (when used consistently and with a definite antecedent), and further reinforce the noun phrase/semantic deep structure property.

The mandatory explicitness of the linguistic elements of coherence links in a basic way the roots of symbolic reference and empirical reference, the latter of which is explicit by nature. To be sure, pro-forms are used for modal reference as well as for empirical reference, but even when pro-forms are used for modal reference, the condition of mandatory explicitness applies, just as the early users of language had to explicitly re-present their empirically-rooted experience. That is, the early users of language initially used language to refer to the here-and-the-now, and from this "symbolic base," they then developed modal reference. We may even go so far as to speculate that the explicit nature of the linguistic elements of is, in the evolutionary sense, a remnant of the explicit nature that all early symbolic reference required. Whether or not this speculation will be proven, we can, through analyses of texts such as those by Halliday and Hasan, Gutwinski, and Markels, attest to the predominantly explicit nature of the linguistic elements as the continuum below demonstrates.

repetition
anaphora
cataphora
ellipsis   ellipsis

Because of the mandatory explicitness of the linguistic elements of coherence, all four categories—repetition, anaphora, cataphora, and ellipsis—are located at the explicit end of the continuum, but because ellipsis has an implicit component, it is also located at the implicit end of the continuum. This continuum will be revised and expanded as chapters three and four explore the explicit and implicit nature of the cohering elements treated in the cognitive and contextually salient perspectives.

CHAPTER THREE

THE COGNITIVE PERSPECTIVE

Basis for the Cognitive Perspective of Coherence

Whereas aspects of the linguistic perspective are frequently and most explicitly manifested in a composition, the aspects of the second perspective of coherence, the cognitive perspective, are often manifested in a liminal manner and serve as a threshold at which distinction between the explicit and implicit blurs. However, the essential bridging effect of these aspects is present in every text. The cognitive perspective is exemplified through such concepts as central cognitive processes, natural semantic domains (i.e., those domains which are not socially constructed but which occur in nature, such as a taxonomy in biology), Gestalt, and the relationship between given and new information. One example from the cognitive perspective is the following text of a very familiar routine:

> (text #1)
> You wake up. You get out of bed. You go to the bathroom. You put on your clothes. You eat. You go to work.

(text #2)
First, you wake up. Then, you get out of bed. Next, you go to the bathroom. After that, you put on your clothes. Then, you eat. Next, you go to work.

(text #3)
You go to the bathroom. You get out of bed. You eat. You wake up. You go to work. You put on your clothes.

(text #4)
First, you go to the bathroom. Then, you get out of bed. Next, you eat. After that, you wake up. Then, you go to work. Next, you put on your clothes.

Members of most cultures or nationalities would find texts #1 and #2 coherent; it is also quite likely that these same persons would have great difficulty in finding text #3 or #4 coherent. (We can note that the explicit logical connectors in text #4 do not render the text coherent.) Text #2 is coherent, and one might posit that such coherence is effected by the logical connectors **first, then, next**, and **after that**. However, one might argue that text #1 is also coherent, without explicit logical connectors such as **first, then, next**, and **after that**.

How then can text #1 be judged coherent?

One response might be that the actions described in text #1 are so familiar as to be almost universal, and indeed that is so. Following this line of argument, text #1 is coherent without the explicit logical connectors employed in text #2 because the actions in text #1 are virtually universal for all humans. However, the actions in text #3 are the very same actions as those in text #1, but text #3 is not coherent. Only the sequence of actions is different, and therein lies the key to the coherence of text #1 and text #2: the SEQUENCE of the actions, i.e., a sequence in time and space that one has come to regard as logical—not the actions alone—enable the coherence of the text. Such a sequence is an example of one of at least fifteen central cognitive processes; other central cognitive processes include but are not limited to contrast, spatializing, comparing, positing causes and/or effects, and classification.

The cognitive perspective is examined through the umbrella concept of the given/new relationship, through Gestalt psychology, and through central cognitive processes, with the intention of identifying elements of the cognitive perspective of coherence and locating these elements on an explicit-implicit continuum.

The Cognitive Perspective of Coherence

The word **cognition** derives from *co* + *gnoscere* (Latin) and *gignoskein* (Greek), meaning to come to know (161). Helpful in the understanding of cognition is the derivation of the related term, **cognate**: *co* + *gnatus* (Latin), to be born; akin to *gignere* (Latin), to beget (161). One additional term will be helpful in understanding what is meant by the cognitive perspective: **cognizance**, which means range of apprehension, of becoming aware (161).

Thus, when one speaks of cognition, one is speaking of purposeful mental activity, and it is precisely this kind of purposeful mental activity a composition teacher seeks to nurture in one's students as they wrestle with and generate their writing.

In a descriptive sense, cognition may be thought of as either unconscious, intuitive, or conscious.

Examples of unconscious cognition are the biochemical threshold and the subconscious. The biochemical threshold deals with the firing of neurons and of the interaction of receptors and synapses, among other neuro-anatomical features. The subconscious deals with aspects such as the id, dreams, repressed thoughts, and pre-intuition.

Intuitive cognition is cognition neither conscious nor unconscious but drawing from and dwelling in both states until the intuition's realization or fruition. It is the "Eureka!" experience which continues to fascinate cognitive scientists and composition teachers alike.

Intuitive cognition may fascinate composition teachers, but it is conscious cognition that these teachers are primarily concerned with. Conscious cognition may be subdivided into unattending and attending cognition. Unattending cognition is cognition in relation to learned behavior which has become virtually automatic. Examples of this are cognition accompanying ordinary speech as in a greeting, the act of checking for traffic before crossing a street, or the habitual setting of an alarm clock.

Attending cognition is cognition that is directed and aware, consciously purposeful (cf. **cognizance**). Attending cognition may be subdivided in the following manner: (1) a normally unattending cognition made attending due to unusual circumstances; (2) metaprocesses;

(3) cogitation. Examples of normally unattending cognition made attending due to unusual circumstances are cognition accompanying the deliberate articulation of an utterance, the crossing of a street with a child for the first several times, or the setting of an alarm at 4:00 a.m. to view Halley's comet. Examples of metaprocesses are thinking about thinking, talking about talking, and so forth. Cogitation, the third subdivision of attending cognition, is the conscious, purposeful use of functional cognitive systems *as* functional cognitive systems. Examples are formal problem solving, the composing of discourse (purposeful use of a symbol system), or a 16-year-old's arguing for the purchase of one's own car. It is this kind of cognition that humans engage in when they consciously and purposefully use functional cognitive systems as functional cognitive systems, whether these systems are a symbol system in the form of written language or the central cognitive processes discussed below.

Cognitive Elements of Coherence

Before examining the concept of central cognitive processes, two other concepts must first be considered, for they to varying degrees subtend all central cognitive processes as well as the linguistic elements of coherence. Those two concepts are the given/new relationship and Gestalt.

The Given/New Relationship

Regardless of one's epistemological foundations or leanings, whether one is an Objectivist, a Cartesian, a Kantian, or whether one hews to the West, to the East, or attempts a synthesis somewhere in between, the given/new relationship is fundamental. Without the given/new relationship, one has no point of orientation (de Beaugrande 184–185): we can only flounder endlessly with no hope of making sense of our thoughts, our environment, or our place in it. A human by nature reasons from given to new. The given is our "old" information, that which we have already been introduced to or stored, and, along with the "new," is fundamentally embedded in epistemological and logical frameworks such as Toulmin's data/warrant/claim, Piaget's assimilation/accommodation, Kuhn's normal science/crisis/revolutionary science, and Hegel's thesis/antithesis/synthesis. Not only does the given orient a person, but it also serves as one's point of departure for cognitive operations, whether the operation is the predication of a sentence, the completion of a hierarchy of categories, or the formation of the categories themselves.

In the prior chapter, four categories of elements in the linguistic perspective of coherence were delineated: repetition, cataphora, anaphora, and ellipsis. All four are subject to the given/new relationship.

Repetition, the duplication of the referent itself, is re-iteration of the given.

[3:1] (G)   (N)   (G) (N) (G)   (N)
He will go home; he will eat; he will sleep.

Cataphora is the reversal of the usual direction of reference: it refers forward from pro-form to referent.

[3:2] (N)   (N)   (G)   (N)
This is what you need to do. You need to go home.

Anaphora represents the normal direction of reference in English, backward from the pro-form to the referent.

[3:3] (G)   (N)   (G)   (N)
John is a good swimmer. He swims three miles daily.

Ellipsis is rarely cataphoric and almost always anaphoric; thus, it, too, is a referring backward from the zero element to the referent, enabled through parallel structure:

[3:4] (G)   (N)   [G] (N)   [G]   (N)
I want to go home, [zero] eat, and [zero] sleep.

What is noteworthy is that the linguistic elements of coherence always represent the given in any particular given/new relationship. This specific property of the linguistic elements helps to explain their mandatory explicitness and their high frequency of occurrence in a text.

Moreover, this relationship to the given illustrates the bond between the relatively few linguistic elements in a text and their maintenance of logical identity in the text. The linguistic elements, by representing the given in a text, ensure a consistent point of reference, thus satisfying what is perhaps the first requisite of coherence.

Not only is the given/new relationship prevalent in the linguistic perspective of coherence as evinced in the above examples, but it is also prevalent in the cognitive perspective as the subsequent discussion of central cognitive processes will show.

Gestalt

The second concept to be considered in the cognitive perspective is Gestalt. As observed in chapter one, humans naturally assume things to "make sense"; "making sense" is the "unmarked" condition or quality of language processing. Coherence is part-and-parcel of normal speech; humans do not communicate not to be understood, but rather to be understood and to understand unless they seek to intentionally obfuscate. This observation is as true of written communication as it is of spoken communication; however, the propensity towards coherence in written communication, especially in extended discourse such as an essay, is offset by the complexities inherent in extended written discourse. Yet these inherent complexities can themselves be offset, at least partly, if one is aware of natural and powerful tendencies in humans which have been studied by Gestalt psychologists.

Gestalt psychologists believe that "organization is basic to all mental activity, that it is unlearned, and that it reflects the way the brain functions" (Gleitman 228). Gestalt may be defined as an "organized whole," a notion clearly akin to the views Aristotle, Horace, and Longinus, as well as contemporary teachers of composition, share regarding the nature of the successful piece of rhetoric. In addition to its focus on the organized whole, Gestalt psychology offers the following concepts which relate closely to the composing process composition teachers emphasize in the classroom: good continuation, closure, and restructuring.

Good continuation is "a powerful organizational factor which will often prevail even when pitted against prior experience" (Gleitman

228–229). An example from nature is the tendency of an observer to view the twigs and branches of a bush as continuations of one another, despite the presence of a praying mantis lodged among the twigs and branches. The observer naturally seeks to view the twigs and branches as continuous parts of the whole bush and quite easily "blends" the slightly discontinuous body of the praying mantis into the body of the bush. Likewise, the composition student, once having completed an outline or rough draft of an essay, will also tend to see a continuity among the various parts of the whole outline or rough draft. Such a tendency can impel the writer to write the outline or the draft despite not yet having all the details at his or her disposal, for the writer "sees" enough of the "twigs or branches" of "the bush" to generate continuity, and ultimately, coherence, for the piece of writing. Or, in other words, good continuation often enables the writer to, as Donald Murray puts it, "glimpse the potential text" (60). Of course, this tendency is two-edged: the student may "see" the continuity when others may not, often due to the outline or rough draft being too "writer-based" and not sufficiently "reader-based" (Flower 19–37).

A second contribution from Gestalt psychology regarding coherence is the principle of closure, defined as the tendency "to complete figures that have gaps in them" (Gleitman 229). If we see only a portion of a circle covered by a card, we will believe that the unseen portion, covered by the card, completes the seen portion, thus making a complete circle.

Likewise, when we see an unfinished sentence or a fill-in-the-blank sentence, we have a tendency to finish the sentence or fill in the blanks. Partly filled-in crossword puzzles also draw on this cognitive tendency toward closure, as does a cloze reading test. Similarly, when we see a "gap" in a draft, we will feel a tendency to close the gap, to make whole, the draft. The challenge for composition teachers, of course, is to instruct the student writers in such a way as for them to "see" the gaps in their drafts so that they will then feel this natural tendency toward closure.

The principle of restructuring is yet another contribution from Gestalt psychology toward an understanding of coherence, especially when the composing process is viewed as an exercise in problem-solving. Gleitman relates that restructuring "involves a dramatic shift in the way [a] problem is viewed.... [T]his shift may be very sudden and is then experienced as a flash of insight, a sense of 'aha' ..." (330). A similar sort of dramatic shift or sense of "aha" occurs when, after wrestling with how to structure a particular piece of discourse or how to frame a particular topic, we finally grasp the structure or the conceptual frame. This particular Gestalt principle is closely associated with the processes involved in creative thinking and hence will be prevalent in those composing situations involving the reflective or emergent thinking that exploratory writing requires (Hairston & Ruszkiewicz 11–12).

Just as the efficient cause was vital to Aristotle's understanding of the nature of knowledge (*Selections* 205), so too is the concept of Gestalt vital to the cognitive perspective of coherence. As Aristotle's efficient cause explains the driving force involved in change or stability, Gestalt entails a natural and powerful "driving force" in humans to relate the part to the whole, and it is this part to whole (or whole to part) relationship which lies at the crux of this approach to coherence, which was defined at the beginning as "the comprehensive, systematic connection of constitutive elements of a text of logical discourse, with a consistent emphasis on both the totality [the whole] of the text and on the interrelatedness of its constituents [its parts]" (chapter one).

Central Cognitive Processes

Central cognitive processes, along with the given/new relationship and the tendency toward Gestalt, are basic to human thought and form a substantial portion of the cognitive universals all humans share. The linguistic elements of coherence, i.e., repetition, anaphora, cataphora, and ellipsis, help maintain logical identity, and the given/new relationship provides a point of logical orientation, but central cognitive processes serve dual purposes, for they are both "pathways" along which humans experience outer and inner reality as well as the "nuts and bolts" humans use as they respond to the Gestalt impetus and attempt to construct satisfactory part to whole and whole to part relationships.

Since classical times, rhetoricians have known of Aristotle's *topoi*, which he viewed as places of the mind and ways of finding something to say (*The Rhetoric* 154). Ross Winterowd uses the concept of a "grammar of coherence" in order to understand better the composing process (828–835). Mary Lawrence, drawing from Jerome Bruner, uses the concept of "structural vocabulary" as a pivot in her approach to composition (5). Randolph Quirk, Sidney Greenbaum, Geoffrey Leech, and Jan Svartvik use the term "logical connecters" (*sic*) to designate numerous logical relationships between clauses (661–676). Rhetorical handbooks use terms such as transitions, modes, thought patterns, and patterns of organization (Bain; Davidson; Hairston & Ruszkiewicz; Corder & Ruszkiewicz). These various terms have in common their recognition of central cognitive processes. Each composition theorist above employs in one's approach central cognitive processes, whether singly, when using a process such as cause and effect, antecedent and consequence, or genus and division, or in combination with other central cognitive processes, as in the expository or argumentative modes.

Central cognitive processes are unique, for they not only occur at the limen on the explicit-implicit continuum of cohering elements, but they also enable humans to generate knowledge as well as organize it. Consequently, central cognitive processes are vital for the invention and arrangement aspects of the composing process and merit special attention.

Jerry Fodor, in *Modularity of Mind*, theorizes about a functional taxonomy of cognition. In his theory, the concept of central systems occupies a key role; the characteristics of these central systems are described below.

> not hardwired/unstable: neuroanatomy
> "relatively diffuse" (118)
>
> quasi assembled: a larger system composed of simpler systems
>
> informationally unencapsulated: central systems access information from each other and from modules
>
> domain neutral: "cut across cognitive domains" (101)
>
> computationally global: may draw on other central systems or modules to perform operations

sensitive to belief system: during computation, central systems consider an individual's set of beliefs

isotropic: confirmation-relevant facts can be "drawn from anywhere in the field of previously established empirical truths" (105)

Quineian: "the degree of confirmation assigned to any given hypothesis is sensitive to properties of the entire belief system; as it were, the shape of our whole science bears on the epistemic status of each scientific hypothesis" (107)

optional engagement: the operation of a central system is not necessarily mandatory;

it can be elective;

variable speed: may be very slow or instantaneous.

These central systems may be thought of as central cognitive processes; that is, central cognitive processes are specific central systems which possess distinguishing characteristics of their own while simultaneously possessing all the characteristics detailed above in Fodor's theory.

Further, these central cognitive processes, as stated earlier, not only guide an individual along "pathways" through and by which one experiences and cogitates outer and inner reality, but they also serve as "nuts and bolts" in the individual's attempts to form coherent views of that which is real in the past and present, and of that which may be possible in the future.

Teachers of composition instruct student writers to go beyond the literal level of language and thought so that they will not only think at the analytic, interpretive, evaluative, and creative levels, but also articulate at these higher levels of thought in coherent essays. Indeed, writing teachers risk being remiss if they do not encourage student writers to look at the underlying logical relationships of the clauses they are connecting and the discourse blocks they are constructing, for this knowledge will give them an increased understanding of how parts of a composition cohere in fundamental, cognitive ways. The characteristics of central systems detailed above—inherent in the central cognitive processes listed below—are those "fundamental, cognitive ways," and it is the central cognitive processes that enable an individual to think in non-linear ways, yet also enable him or her to attempt to express non-linear thought within the constraints of linear language.

While our expressions in language are constrained by linearity, our thinking and mental imagery are not (chapter two). A significant feature of central cognitive processes, and to a lesser degree, of the given/new relationship and of Gestalt, is their inherent capacity for enabling non-linear thought. Waldron relates that the leap from sign to symbol is monumental because symbolic reference is itself a multi-faceted cognitive operation (50).

When we use a linguistic symbol, we not only assign a label to an entity, thus employing a referential function to the symbol, but we also assign to the symbol a logical identity by which we distinguish it from other items, thus employing a differential function; as we differentiate between referents, we naturally form categories; thus, the use of a linguistic symbol is also the beginning of the categorial function, and categorization entails central cognitive processes such as contrast, comparison, classification, and hierarchiazation.

Language and higher thought, then, truly develop *pari passu*, for to use the linguistic symbol is to immediately engage fundamental and powerful cognitive systems, and yet without the linguistic symbol, these same cognitive systems would be inexpressible.

Thus, the listing below of central cognitive processes as elements in the cognitive perspective of coherence is also the listing of powerful processes that cut across cognitive domains, processes that are not just inter-connected, but which are isotropic. They are also processes that access long-term and short-term memory, that are engaged at the option of the individual person, and that may be used at a speed dependent on the discretion of the individual.

These central cognitive processes are listed in a developmental continuum, along with illustrative examples and explicit markers. The developmental continuum is tentative, but it may be seen as a provisional step toward understanding how one central cognitive process is logically prior to another. Jung argues that "differentiation is the essence, the *sine qua non* of consciousness" (95). Contrast, then, may be thought of as a primal cognitive act; it could first occur when a baby finally becomes aware of the me/not me distinction regarding its body and the rest of its world. Such a distinction is used by Edmund Leach in elaborating the notion of binary coding, a property which, he argues, is common to human communication (62–63). Further, if categorizing is defined as grouping by differences or similarities, then both contrasting and comparing must be logically prior to categorizing. Similarly, if hierarchizing is seen as an ordering of categories according to levels of subordination or superordination, then contrasting, comparing, and categorizing are logically prior to it.

Likewise, analogizing presumes contrasting and comparing, at the very least, because it consists of drawing parallels or similarities between or among dissimilar entities. However, such entities may also be hierarchies themselves, and thus analogizing presumes hierarchiazation, as well as contrast, comparison, and analogy. Synthesizing, defined as the expressing of coherence among seemingly disparate entities or relationships, is listed in the final position because when we synthesize, we are free to draw on any combination of the other central cognitive processes in order to express such a coherence.

Below is a detailed list of these central cognitive processes, their rendering either implicitly or explicitly, as well as their explicit markers:

[3:5] CONTRASTING: the indicating of differences between

> implicit rendering:
>
>> Thomas Jefferson was a very orderly and temperate man; Samuel Adams was absent-minded and hot-tempered.
>
> explicit rendering:
>
>> Thomas Jefferson was a very orderly and temperate man, **unlike** Samuel Adams, who was absent-minded and hot-tempered.
>
> explicit markers:
>
>> on the contrary, by comparison, on the one hand ... on the other hand, by way of contrast, instead, but, although, however, differ

from, different from, still, otherwise, even so, nevertheless, still, dissimilarly, less than, more than, faster than (etc.), in contrast, in opposition, on the opposite side, while, admittedly, in reality, of course, actually, true

[3:6] SPATIALIZING: the ordering of items in space

implicit rendering: none possible

explicit rendering: Please place the green chair **here**, the red one **there**, and the couch in **between**.

explicit markers:

next to, alongside of, in, into, out of, outside of, over, under, underneath, below, above, across, among, around, before, behind, beneath, beside, beyond, off, opposite, round, through, within, north, south, east, west, to the right, to the left, front, middle, rear, side, adjacent midpoint, endpoint, diagonal, edge, parallel, perpendicular, co-planar, overlapping, vertical, horizontal

[3:7] COMPARING: the indicating of similarities between entities

implicit rendering:

Jefferson believed passionately in freedom of thought and freedom of religion. Franklin, another "founding father," believed strongly in freedom of thought and freedom of religion.

explicit rendering:

Jefferson believed passionately in freedom of thought and freedom of religion. **So, too,** did Franklin.

explicit markers:

as, just as, similarly, similar to, in the same way, almost the same, at the same rate as, like, alike, likewise, in like manner, correspond to, correspondingly, resemble, resemblance, to be parallel in ... , to have ... in common, common features, characteristics, etc.

[3:8] POSITING CAUSE AND EFFECT: the stating of an action or a condition and its result

implicit rendering:

Unfortunately, John went out drinking last night. He drove recklessly. Now, he is in the hospital, paralyzed from the waist down.

explicit rendering:

> Unfortunately, John went out drinking last night. **Because** he did so, he drove recklessly. Now, as a tragic **consequence**, he is in the hospital, paralyzed from the waist down.

explicit markers:

> so, so that, so much (so) that, thus, consequently, as a consequence, in consequence, therefore, accordingly, for, for fear (that), for the purpose that, for this reason, as a result, hence, because, because of, owing to, since, due to, being that, in that, in the hope that, seeing that, so much that, inasmuch as, forasmuch as, in view of, with this in mind, with this intention, to the end that, lest, if, even if, only if, unless, in case, provided that, providing that, on (the) condition that, in the event that given that, granted (that), granting (that), as long as, so long as, then, if so, in that case, that being the case, under those circumstances, if not, otherwise

[3:9] CATEGORIZING: grouping by similarities or differences

implicit rendering:

> Apples, oranges, and tangerines contain seeds. Fish, beef, and mutton are meats.

explicit rendering:

> Apples, oranges, and tangerines are **alike** in that they **all** contain seeds. Fish, beef, and mutton are **similar** in that they **all** are meats.

explicit markers:

> as, just as, similarly, similar to, in the same way, almost the same, at the same rate as, like, alike, likewise, in like manner, correspond to, correspondingly, resemble, resemblance, to be parallel in ... , to have ... in common, common features, characteristics, etc., on the contrary, instead, by comparison, on the one hand ... on the other hand, by way of contrast, but, although, however, differ from, different from, still, otherwise, even so, nevertheless, still, dissimilarly, less than, more than, faster than (etc.), in contrast, in opposition, on the opposite side, while, admittedly, in reality, of course, actually, true

THE COGNITIVE PERSPECTIVE 51

[3:10] SPECIFYING: the providing of a detail at a lower level of generalization for an entity at a greater level of generalization

implicit rendering:

Diogenes was a simple man. His only material possessions were his toga and a bowl.

explicit rendering:

Diogenes was a simple man. **For example**, his only material possessions were his toga and a bowl.

explicit markers:

for example, for instance, for one thing, to illustrate, in one instance, in other words, as follows, as proof, let me illustrate, let me cite as proof, in substantiation, to substantiate, as an illustration, in this instance, as an example, in practice, according to statistics, according to statistical evidence, such as, especially, particularly, in particular, notably, by way of example, namely, to be specific, specifically, that is (to say); take ... , for example; consider ... , for example

[3:11] ANALYZING: the stating of component parts

implicit rendering: none possible

explicit rendering:

Although now regarded by many as a quaint form of transportation, a bicycle **consists of** several highly-tooled **parts, including** tires, rims, spokes, a chain, and cables.

explicit markers:

consists of, is composed of, divides into, includes, including, have, has, components, parts, aspects, qualities, attributes, characteristics, factors, eras, times, regions, sector, factor, piece, particle, section, member, segment, constituent, element, ingredient, feature, contents

[3:12] INDUCING: the drawing of a conclusion from particulars

implicit rendering:

Holmes turned to Watson. "The chemical tests confirm that Eggert's hands carried sulphur. Eggert was at the scene of the crime. And he has sufficient motive.""Eggert is our man!" exclaimed Watson." Holmes only furrowed his brow and said, "Perhaps."

explicit rendering:

> Holmes turned to Watson. "The chemical tests confirm that Eggert's hands carried sulphur. Eggert was at the scene of the crime. And he has sufficient motive. ""**Therefore** Eggert is our man!" exclaimed Watson. " Holmes only furrowed his brow and said, "Perhaps."

explicit markers:

> so, thus, consequently, therefore, accordingly, for these reasons, as a result, hence, because, because of, owing to, since, due to, it follows, being that, seeing that, as, inasmuch as, in view of, owing to

[3:13] CHRONOLOGIZING: the ordering of entities according to time

implicit rendering:

> He unlocked the door and entered the dark room. He turned on the lights. The room erupted in shouts and huzzahs of celebration.

explicit rendering:

> **First**, he unlocked the door and entered the dark room. **Next**, he turned on the lights. **Then**, the room erupted in shouts and huzzahs of celebration.

explicit markers:

> then, now, nowadays, at the present, when, before, after, while, during, between ... and ... , in (month/year), in the (period of the day, e.g., morning, afternoon), on (day of week or date), since ..., later, earlier, formerly every (number) (years, months, days, minutes, etc.), at the turn of the century (decade, etc.), in the first (second, etc.) part of the century (month, week, day, etc.), in the 1800s, etc., at birth, in childhood, in infancy, in adolescence, as an adult, in adulthood, in old age, at death, simultaneously, simultaneous with, at the same time as, contemporaneously, co-eval, former, latter, previous, previously, prior to, first, second, etc., in the first place, in the second place, etc., to begin with, to end with, next, subsequently, at last, in conclusion, finally

[3:14] GENERALIZING: the stating of a principle based upon specific observations

implicit rendering:

> Rafe is only seven years old; he did not realize he was plagiarizing Lincoln. Olivia is only three years old; she did not know that it

is wrong to take cookies without asking. Children are innocent in things such as these.

explicit rendering:

Rafe is only seven years old; he did not realize he was plagiarizing Lincoln. Olivia is only three years old; she did not know that it is wrong to take cookies without asking. **All** children are innocent in things such as these.

explicit markers:

generally, generally speaking, on the whole, all, every, never, always

[3:15] HIERARCHIAZATION: the classifying of categories

implicit rendering: none possible

explicit rendering:

American government can be **subdivided** into four **levels**: local, county, state, and national. **Each** of these **consists** of branches **comprised** of **subordinate** departments, bureaus, and ministries.

explicit markers:

classified, subdivided, levels, graded, sorted, ranked, arranged, ordered, organized, stratified, bracketed, codified, lower, higher, consists of, is composed of, divides into, includes, including, have, has, components, parts, aspects, qualities, attributes, characteristics, factors, eras, times, regions, sector, factor, piece, particle, section, member, segment, constituent, element, ingredient, feature, contents, each, every, single, respective

[3:16] DEDUCING: the drawing of a conclusion by reasoning from a generality

implicit rendering:

All her brothers have big feet, pale skin, and light eyes. Hans has big feet, pale skin, and light eyes. Hans is her brother.

explicit rendering:

All have big feet, pale skin, and light eyes. Hans has big feet, pale skin, and light eyes. **Consequently**, Hans is her brother.

explicit markers:

generally, generally speaking, on the whole, all, every, never, always so, so that, so much (so) that, thus, consequently, as a consequence, in consequence, therefore accordingly, for, for fear (that), for the purpose that, for this reason, as a result, hence, because, because of, owing to, since, due to, being that, in that, in the hope that, seeing that, so much that, inasmuch as, forasmuch as, in view of, with this in mind, with this intention, to the end that, lest, if, even if, only if, unless, in case, provided that, providing that, on (the) conditions that, in the event that given that, granted (that), granting (that), as long as, so long as, then, if so, in that case, that being the case, under those circumstances, if not, otherwise

[3:17] ABSTRACTING: the assigning of a quality or an intangible to an entity, often tangible

implicit rendering:

>Daily, she sacrifices for the poor. Hourly, she prays for the lost. By the minute, she toils to heal the sick. Mother Theresa is love.

explicit rendering:

>Daily, she sacrifices for the poor. Hourly, she prays for the lost. By the minute, she toils to heal the sick. **In essence**, Mother Theresa is love.

explicit markers:

>in essence, essentially, in a word, quintessentially, obviously, clearly, without a doubt, nothing but, sheer, pure, purely

[3:18] HYPOTHESIZING: the stating of a possible explanation or of a contingent relationship

implicit rendering: none possible

explicit rendering:

>**If** Noble Banadda **had** not succumbed to Covid, he surely **would have** made even more of a mark on science (Noble Banadda; Tuhereze).

explicit markers:

>if ... then, if so, had, should, in (that) case, provided that, providing that, on the condition that, in the event that, given that, granted (that), granting (that) as long as, so long as, even if, only if, that being

the case, under those circumstances, unless, if not, otherwise; were, would, and other subjunctive renderings

[3:19] ANALOGIZING: the expressing of similarity between or among dissimilar entities or relationships

implicit rendering:

The successful actor can perform on the stage in a variety of roles. The successful person can function well in a number of positions.

explicit rendering:

Just as the successful actor can perform on the stage in a variety of roles, **so too** can the successful person function well in a number of positions.

explicit markers:

analogously, as, just as, similarly, similar to, in the same way, almost the same, like, alike, likewise, in like manner, correspond to, correspondingly, resemble, resemblance, to be parallel in ... , to have ... in common, common features, characteristics, etc.

[3:20] SYNTHESIZING: this, the paramount central cognitive process, transcend analogy and engages all other central cognitive processes to express coherence among seemingly disparate entities

implicit rendering:

Hydrogen is a plentiful yet explosive gas. Mercury is a shiny and toxic liquid quite sensitive to temperatures. Iron is a hard and somewhat brittle solid which decomposes when exposed to air and water. They are fundamental substances called elements and cannot be decomposed into other substances.

explicit rendering:

Hydrogen is a plentiful yet explosive gas. Mercury is a shiny and toxic liquid quite sensitive to temperature. Iron is a hard and somewhat brittle solid which decomposes when exposed to air and water. **However different** they may be superficially, **all three share** a unique characteristic. They are fundamental substances called elements and cannot be decomposed into other substances.

explicit markers:

> the central cognitive process of synthesis is explicitly rendered using explicit markers from any of the other central cognitive processes

The purpose of the list, then, is not to establish its inclusiveness, but to embrace under a single rubric such concepts as Aristotle's *topoi*, Winterowd's grammar of coherence, Lawrence's structural vocabulary, Quirk, Greenbaum, Leech, and Svartik's logical connecters, and terms often used in handbooks or within the discipline such as transitions, modes, thought patterns, and patterns of organization.

The central cognitive processes occupy the limen portion of the continuum below because of the variable nature of their overt markers; at times, their overt markers are necessary, but often they are optional, depending on the rhetorical situation.

An Explicit-Implicit Continuum

Our treatment of the linguistic perspective of coherence (chapter two) resulted in the continuum below:

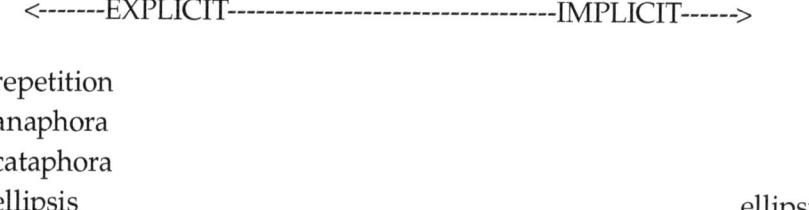

<-------EXPLICIT----------------------------------IMPLICIT----->

repetition
anaphora
cataphora
ellipsis   ellipsis

We noted that because of the mandatory explicitness of the linguistic elements of coherence, all four categories—repetition, anaphora, cataphora, and ellipsis—are located at the explicit end of the continuum, but because ellipsis has an implicit component, it is also located at the implicit end of the continuum.

We also noted that the linguistic elements of coherence have special properties which serve an essential role in the cohering of discourse, and that among these properties are their dominant word form, their small number and high frequency in a text, their representing the given in the given/new relationship, and their mandatory explicitness.

Just as the linguistic elements have special properties which serve to enable coherence, so too do the cognitive elements of coherence. Paramount among these is the property of parallel distributed processing. This property accounts for the interconnection of the above listed central cognitive processes across domains, thus affording a second property the significance of which is difficult to overestimate: utility. If the linguistic elements of coherence perform a vital function by maintaining the identity of the given in any particular given/new relationship, the cognitive elements of coherence enables us to consummate the given/new relationship by allowing us to bring to it the "new" constituent or to fashion any logical relationship, be it one of contrast, analysis, or analogy. Further, the versatility of central cognitive processes enables an individual to do this at the level of clause, paragraph, essay, or book, at the micro-state or at the macro-state, depending on the degree of chunking. Chapter four will deal with the contextual salience perspective of coherence and demonstrate that not only do humans use central cognitive processes at various levels, but they also use them in various combinations, depending on their purpose and on specific elements of contextual salience.

Unlike the linguistic elements of coherence, which always have a mandatory explicit component manifested in the text through and by language expressly for co-referential purposes, the cognitive elements of coherence may be manifested in a liminal manner and serve as a threshold at which the explicit/implicit distinction blurs, as in the case of the central cognitive processes. Or, a cognitive element may be explicit, witness the given/new relationship. Cognitive elements may also be entirely implicit, as in the case of the elements deriving from Gestalt psychology: good continuation, closure, and restructuring.

Consequently, the explicit-implicit continuum, with elements coded from both the **linguistic** and *cognitive* perspectives of coherence, approximates the following:

```
<-------EXPLICIT-------------limen---------------IMPLICIT------>
```

given/new relationship   *good continuation*
                                         closure
                                         restructuring

                         central
                         cognitive
repetition   *processes*
anaphora
cataphora
ellipsis   **ellipsis**

The given/new relationship enables humans to have a point of orientation (de Beaugrande 184–185) in their reasoning and forms, along with co-reference and logical identity, the nucleus of natural language logic. The elements of Gestalt—good continuation, closure, and restructuring—provide the impetus to humans for reasoning from part to whole and whole to part. Central cognitive processes are universal to humans, operate freely across all cognitive domains, and process information in a parallel, distributed fashion. They enable humans to not only generate thought, but to organize it. Thus, the elements of the cognitive perspective are vital to coherence. Consequently, they possess a unique value in the composition classroom.

CHAPTER FOUR

THE CONTEXTUALLY SALIENT PERSPECTIVE

Basis for the Contextually Salient Perspective of Coherence

The third perspective of coherence, that of contextual salience, is usually manifested in the text through such implied but powerful, fundamental, and culturally-related concepts as epistemological frames, central metaphors, sociological models, and warrants.

The following example illustrates how contextual salience, or, in this case, subcultural salience, dramatically affects coherence through the lexicon:

> When the tool locates the object, he may name that location to the stalls, saying in an undertone "left bridge" or "right bridge" or "kiss the dog," or whatever instructions may be necessary to inform the stalls, so that they can put the patient into position for the tool to operate. The tool may likewise communicate with the stalls during the operation, giving them instructions such as "roust" or "come through," or "stick," or "stick and split me out" or "turn him for a pit," etc. All tools give the stalls an office or signal when they remove the object... . To this researcher "it seems incredible" that the patient does not realize that the language is focused almost exclusively on him. (Adapted from Maurer 53–54)

Here is evinced one prominent part of the context, the subculture, implicit and not mentioned in the text, but which makes salient a specific semantic domain manifested explicitly in the text via a specialized vocabulary. Such specialized vocabulary is an essential element of the coherence of this particular text, and the explicit-implicit relationship between specialized vocabulary representing semantic domains and the subculture also holds for entire texts written across the curriculum, whether in business, law, science, technology, or the arts.

The earlier passage from *Alice in Wonderland* indicates that the linguistic elements of coherence are the elements used the most frequently and the most explicitly. Similarly, the passage describing the early morning routine and its sequence of familiar actions illustrates how the cognitive elements of coherence serve bridging or liminal functions, at times explicit and at times implicit. In like manner, the above passage using the *argot* of pickpockets illustrates that the elements of the contextually salient perspective rely on culturally-related concepts such as epistemological frames, central metaphors, sociological metaphors, and warrants.

Most humans strive to make sense of life, to discover a coherence in, if not of, life. History and literature are replete with humans engaged in this quest, from figures of note such as Solomon, laden with riches and satiated with pleasures, who continued to quest for coherence in life as recorded in Ecclesiastes and much of Proverbs, to the "small" characters in Tolstoy's *War and Peace* and *Anna Karenina*, and those of Dostoevsky in *The Brothers Karamazov, Crime and Punishment,* and *The Idiot*, who from their inauspicious beginnings and endings raise the enduring questions of love and hate, justice and injustice, of faith in and doubts of life itself. Regardless of their station in life, these characters wrestle with and through language in their quest for coherence. Language is indispensable in this quest. As Knoblauch and Brannon tell us,

> Modern rhetorical theory, beginning as early as the seventeenth century, finds a closer connection between language and thought, discourse and knowledge, than ancient speculation had supposed. Far from serving an

optional, ceremonial function, composition—the forming process at the heart of writing—is essentially related to learning, to the individual's personal search for coherence in experience. It is also, as a manifestation of human symbolic capacities, a natural endowment in essence, not a technical skill. (4)

In this quest for coherence, then, humans use "the natural endowment" of language, whether in life in general or in a composition class in particular.

E. D. Hirsch, Jr., maintains that "the peculiar nature of coherence ... is not an absolute, but a dependent quality" (237). He goes on to argue that

> The laws of coherence are variable; they depend upon the nature of the total meaning under consideration. Two meanings ("dark" and "bright," for example) which cohere in one context may not cohere in another. "Dark with excessive bright" makes excellent sense in *Paradise Lost*, but if a reader found the passage in a textbook on plant pathology, he would assume that he confronted a misprint for "Dark with excessive blight." Coherence depends on the context, and it is helpful to recall our definition of context: it is a sense of the whole meaning, constituted of explicit partial meanings plus a horizon of expectations and probabilities. (237)

Or, as Patricia Carrell puts it, "processing a text is an interactive process between the text and the background knowledge or memory schemata of the listener or reader. In the schema-theoretical view of text processing, what is important is not only text, its structure and content, but what the reader or listener does with text" (482). I hasten to add that for the purposes of this theory toward coherence, the interactive process includes not only listening and reading, but also speaking and writing.

Traditionally, the surface language of a text has been the focus for the analysis of coherence. In actuality, however, the surface language of a text does not bear all the burden of achieving coherence, as the implicit nature of some of the central cognitive processes illustrates. Consequently, the scope of this work includes the contextually salient perspective as well as the linguistic and cognitive perspectives. By considering implicit elements as well as explicit ones, we can more accurately represent how various elements of a text contribute to the coherence of a composition or essay.

While the linguistic elements of coherence may be used the most frequently and the most explicitly in the text of a composition or essay, and the cognitive elements of coherence serve bridging or liminal functions, at times explicit and at times implicit, elements of the contextually salient perspective are manifested in the text through implied but powerful, fundamental, and culturally-related concepts such as epistemological frames, central metaphors, sociological models, and warrants.

Because the contextually salient perspective of coherence is culturally related, it often seems to be omnipresent and ubiquitous. Paradoxically, it is often the most implicit aspect of coherence, seldom manifesting itself explicitly or directly through language meant to be understood at the literal level, as in the linguistic and cognitive categories. As Jerry Won Lee tells us, "communication need not be treated as limited to 'language' but as inviting attention to the wide range of semiotic resources and spatial elements that are constitutive of a communicative moment or phenomena" (31). So, regardless of the culture—or cultures—involved in the communication, regardless of the cultured-ness of one interlocutor or another, in each instance of linguistic communication a whole range of factors is at play, and as Lee argues, such expression can be an opportunity to recognize not just the explicit, often taken-for-granted aspects of the communication, but also the implicit and sometimes very subtle aspects of the communication. It is these latter aspects that are part-and-parcel of the culturally salient perspective of coherence.

Thus, elements of the contextually salient perspective manifest themselves in language meant to be understood at the interpretive level in the form of word choice, grammatical structure (voice, nominalizations, etc.), rhetorical pattern of sentences, thesis placement, and prevalence of particular central cognitive processes, often resulting in emphasis on a particular arrangement or pattern of thought. The following overview of the contextually salient perspective will examine the interrelationships of epistemological frames, central metaphors, sociological models, and warrants as they serve to enable the coherence of a text.

The Contextually Salient Perspective of Coherence

Epistemology deals with how humans know what they know and what they accept as sensible and logical, and hence, what they view as coherent. A human's epistemological framework, then, subtends and permeates all his or her other logical relationships and operations.

In the West, two main epistemological frameworks have evolved, *die Geisteswissenschaften* (the humanities) and *die Naturwissenschaften* (the natural sciences) (Dilthey). Die Geisteswissenschaften is an inclusive framework which accords equal epistemological status to intangible entities such as thoughts, ideas, abstractions, dreams, and logical relationships, as well as to tangible entities such as those represented by one or more of the senses of sight, sound, touch, taste, and smell. Die Naturwissenschaften is an exclusive framework which accords greater epistemological status to tangible data, ostensibly accepting as valid only that which has empirical characteristics. Another key distinction made between these two dominant frameworks is that die Geisteswissenschaften is essentially retrodictive and die Naturwissenschaften is essentially predictive.

The consequences of epistemological frames are apparent. For example, the seminarian operating from the premises of Naturwissenschaften will likely encounter much difficulty, just as the behavioral psychologist who admits only empirical data will meet with frustration. In effect, the epistemological frame serves as a filter for what may be considered logical. Thus, an epistemological frame influences our lives in the most fundamental of ways. It determines our very view of reality and the manner by which we deal with this reality. An epistemological frame, then, determines what is sensible and logical, and thus, what is coherent for an individual.

Central Metaphors

In 1980, George Lakoff and Mark Johnson wrote *In Metaphors We Live By* that metaphors have traditionally been viewed in philosophy and linguistics as "a matter of peripheral interest" (ix). However, Lakoff and Johnson provide copious linguistic evidence which refutes this "peripheral" view. Indeed, they argue convincingly that "metaphor is pervasive in everyday language and thought" (ix) and that metaphor is "as much a part of our functioning as our sense of touch" (239). This work in coherence theory follows this same argument. Consequently, metaphor comprises the second element examined in the contextually salient perspective.

Metaphor is defined as a type of one of the central cognitive processes, analogy. Metaphor consists of two pairs of elements; one half of each pair, called the attributant, expresses qualities or characteristics. The remaining half of each pair has a naming function and is called the nominal. These terms are used because they are discipline neutral and functional in nature, as opposed to those common to literary criticism such as tenor, vehicle, and image, which presuppose a theory of tension in treating metaphor (Richards 1936). Instead, the relationship used here emphasizes a mapping between cognitive domains.

Consider the following four metaphorical expressions: (A) That boxer is a tiger; (B) **Hought** is pronounced so that it rhymes with **bought**; (C) The world is a stage; (D) School is incarceration.

Metaphor A may be thought of as consisting of the following two pairs of elements:

elemental pair 1 for Metaphor A:
animal with great strength & quickness (attributant)
tiger (nominal)
elemental pair 2 for Metaphor A:
man with great strength & quickness (attributant)
boxer (nominal)
Metaphor A => That boxer is a tiger.

Metaphor B (Glass, Holyoak, & Santa 1979) may be thought of as consisting of the following two pairs of elements:

elemental pair 1 for Metaphor B:
familiar consonant cluster/known pronunciation (attributant)
bought (nominal)
elemental pair 2 for Metaphor B:
familiar consonant cluster/unknown pronunciation (attributant)

hought (nominal)
Metaphor B => **Hought** rhymes with **bought**.

Metaphor C may be thought of as consisting of the following pairs of elements:

elemental pair 1 for Metaphor C:
the place where actors roleplay (attributant)
stage (nominal)
elemental pair 2 for Metaphor C:
the place where humans function in various roles (attributant)
unknown life model (nominal)
Metaphor C => The world is a stage.

Metaphor D may be thought of as consisting of the following pairs of elements:

elemental pair 1 for Metaphor D:
institution with armed guards, searches, and lockdowns (attributant)
place of incarceration (nominal)
elemental pair 2 for Metaphor D:
school with armed guards, searches, and lockdowns (attributant)
school (nominal)
Metaphor D => School is incarceration. (Everett 45–47)

All metaphors derive from two elemental pairs. Of the four elements (two attributants and two nominals), at least three must be known. Of the three known elements, cognitive focus is on the two parallel elements, either attributant:attributant or nominal:nominal.

Further, any number of the central cognitive processes subsumed by analogy can be utilized in order to achieve the metaphor (cf. chapter three). Hence, the emphasis is on a mapping between cognitive domains rather than on a theory of tension as seen in literary analysis.

Such mapping between cognitive domains occurs when we use a metaphor as a device for the bridging of linguistic, cognitive, and experiential gaps. Linguistic bridging occurs when one has the thoughts and the commonality of experience, but not the language, due to a deficit in the speaker's idiolect or in the language itself: for example, a speaker of English who, failing to find the adequate language in one's native tongue, resorts to a Japanese proverb which uses metaphor: "The hungry dog does not fear the stick" (De Lange 34). Cognitive bridging occurs when one cannot apprehend meaning despite adequate language and commonality of experience: for example, we may use the hand as metaphor to explain the concept of base ten in mathematics. Experiential bridging occurs when one cannot apprehend meaning despite adequate language and cognition: for example, an extra-terrestrial's borrowing from Earth culture a metaphor in order to explain to an Earthling a circumstance peculiar to the extra-terrestrial's world.

A metaphor may also serve as an expressive device, the kind of which is often used in poetry, colorful language, or literature:

> That boxer is a tiger!
>
> or
>
> Or ever the silver cord is loosed, or the golden bowl is broken, or the pitcher is broken at the fountain, or the wheel broken at the cistern; Then shall the dust return to the earth as it was, and the spirit shall return unto God, who gave it. (Ecclesiastes 12:6–7)

A metaphor may also serve as a condensed expression: for example, in answer to the question "What kind of politician was Margaret Thatcher?" one replies "She was a female version of Ronald Reagan, but more cerebral and candid."

Thus, metaphor is a much-used central cognitive process; we often use a metaphor as we attempt to explain to others or to our inner selves how one aspect of reality relates to another. Weighty expressions such as "life is a journey" or "the world is a stage" and less weighty expressions such as "that boxer is a tiger" or "she's a trip" help us communicate and understand what we think or feel.

Accordingly, a tendency towards a wide use of metaphor seems second nature, and rarely do we shy from it; rather, more often than not, when a particular metaphor fails, we search with alacrity for other metaphors that might better convey our understanding. We might think "X is like Y—no, like Z! No, X is like A! Yes, that's it! X *is* A!" However, of the many metaphors we humans employ daily and hourly to help us better communicate or understand, we, in a desire to simplify life and our comprehension of it, often employ a metaphor which subsumes all other metaphors, and indeed, permeates our thoughts and emotions and either reinforces our instincts or conflicts with them. Such a metaphor may be called a central metaphor.

A central metaphor serves humans in two crucial ways, as guide and as touchstone. A central metaphor serves as guide when it indicates to us our role, and consequently, our behavior, in life. Just as importantly, a central metaphor also serves as guide when it indicates the role and behavior we come to expect from fellow humans and from our environment. A central metaphor serves as touchstone when we return to it to reassure ourselves of our own world view and to re-affirm concord with our epistemological frame. In a sense, it serves as a place in our consciousness where we can always go in order to sort out the variables and changes of life. Central metaphors, then, are of the utmost importance in life.

Because they serve as shorthand versions of epistemological frames, their number is few, and we normally use an even smaller—and consistent—number of them, for they must be reasonably consistent not only with our epistemological frame, but also with our belief system. Some individuals may embrace the central metaphor of games and compete in a more-or-less happy fashion according to an agreed-upon set of rules for designated prizes. Other individuals—less fortunate—may choose to die before exchanging particular central metaphors. Witness the individual who has embraced the central metaphor of chance and uses it as an excuse to continue an addiction to alcohol or to gambling (Brown). Thus, central metaphors are quite powerful and exert great influence on individuals.

In chapter three, we saw that central cognitive processes are isotropic and sensitive to belief systems. Central metaphors are particularly isotropic and sensitive to belief systems. Whenever we seek to apply or validate a specific central metaphor, we are utilizing the central cognitive process of analogy, and due to its position in the hierarchy of all central cognitive processes, we may employ any of the subsumed central cognitive processes (only the central cognitive process of synthesis is not subsumed by analogy). Further, because of the isotropic quality of central cognitive processes, we can draw from "anywhere in the field of previously established empirical truths" to confirm that a configuration of data is indeed what it seems to be (Fodor 105). For example, in order for us to use the central cognitive process of classification to determine that the object that a set of adjectives is describing is a college professor, one may draw from any of one's empirical experiences to confirm that the object is actually a college professor.

However, central cognitive processes, and by extension, central metaphors, are not limited to empirical data, for, as Fodor argues, they are also sensitive to one's belief system. For example, if a prosperous, white individual were to see an African-American male on his way to a predominantly African-American high school in a depressed neighborhood, the individual could easily believe that that young man would eventually end up in prison, when in fact, the high school student was actually a high achiever, making excellent grades in school, scoring in the ninetieth percentiles on national exams, was a member of the mayor's youth advisory council, and had never had any sort of problems with the police (Everett 35). As Canagarajah tells us in "Weaving the Text: Changing Literacy Practices and Orientations," this is an example of how "some interlocutors may refuse to adopt the code of cross-cultural conduct or impose their own norms" (16).

So we see that not only are individual central cognitive processes sensitive to one's belief system in the intra-cultural sense, but also in the cross-cultural sense. Moreover, dominant thought patterns can vary from culture to culture (see Kameda for work on the Japanese dominant thought pattern, Qin for the Chinese, Montaño-Harmon for the Mexican, and Kaplan for an earlier view of thought patterns across various cultures). Thus, the belief systems of the individual and of the individual's culture influence significantly what and how data are classified, hypothesized, abstracted, and analogized, as well as whether the dominant arrangement in a text is of one particular order or another. If the data are not processed or arranged in accordance with the belief system, the result is judged incongruous with one's central metaphor, and quite possibly, incoherent.

Accordingly, Lakoff argues that metaphors go beyond the traditional view of figures of speech (tropes): metaphors are "figures of thought"

(215). This view more accurately reflects the variety of elements and immense scope of central metaphors; however, it also reveals the complexity of central metaphors for the following reasons:

(1) All thought ultimately derives from time and space relations, and it is arguable that time is a function of space, or at the very least, is dependent upon space for its conceptualization (Jones 77–83).
(2) Central metaphors are ubiquitous: they exist in unconscious as well as conscious cognition, and they may be instrumental in certain instances of intuition. Further, central metaphors, because they are metaphors, are a type of analogy, the central cognitive process which subsumes all other central cognitive processes except that of synthesis, and as a central cognitive process, is, among other characteristics, domain neutral and isotropic.
(3) Metaphors, due to their position in the hierarchy of central cognitive processes, are isotropic to a very great degree, and the greater the isotropism, the less one can comprehend the process (Fodor 106); this property is intensified in a central metaphor because of its scope.

Metaphor, then, is limited only by space and its relationship in the hierarchy of central cognitive processes: consequently, central metaphors overarch one's thought processes and exert tremendous power and influence in one's perception of how various elements of perceived reality interrelate; indeed, central metaphors determine these very relationships.

The following are categories of some of the more dominant central metaphors: the metaphor of growth, which has its formal roots in classical Greek thought and is seen in various guises, for example, as process or progress; the metaphor of drama, in which life is viewed as a stage and members of society perform various roles; the metaphor of chance, in which life is likened to a game of chance or fortune; the metaphor of games, in which members of society compete according to an agreed-upon set of rules for designated prizes (Brown).

These and other central metaphors subtend virtually all the aspects of one's consciousness and thus, one's notion of what fits with what, what makes sense, what does not, and, significantly, what serves to enable coherence and what does not.

Because of their powerful and deep influence, central metaphors lead to the formulation of sociological models, through and by which humans conduct their lives. All the sociological models sketched below "assume that human beings negotiate their way through life in quest for meaning" (St. Clair, "Language" 225), and that language is the medium of symbolic representation which humans use for the construction or understanding of social reality and the maintenance of cultural values; further, language is the medium of symbolic representation for an individual, a group, or a society as problems, topics, or questions of self and society are explored in a quest for coherence. Within each of the four models of sociology outlined below, language is used in various ways as an individual engages in interpretive, analytical, critical, and creative thought, going beyond the level of signs, of surface impressions, and surface thinking. In so doing, the individual consciously and purposively uses language as a symbol system in an attempt to form or fit one's developing knowledge into a coherent whole.

This treatment of central metaphors and sociological models does not imply that an individual will employ a fixed number of central metaphors and a particular sociological model and only those metaphors and model, although this may be the case in some instances. Rather, this treatment seeks to reveal how individuals may use various central metaphors and sociological models, including but not limited to those mentioned below. Some individuals may vary their operative central metaphors and sociological models as circumstances dictate.

Sociological Models

Each of the two larger divisions of sociological models— symbolic interactionism and phenomenology—embodies the notion of social construction. Symbolic interactionism embodies the concept of a socially constructed world; phenomenology embodies the construction of social consciousness. Whether the sociological model is one of symbolic interactionism or of phenomenology, it may be subtended by a single central metaphor or a small number of central metaphors which act as a core of *ad hoc* epistemological frames which help an individual negotiate his or her way through life in some sort of coherent manner. For example, if we embrace the central metaphor that "all the world is a stage" and we have roles in which we should perform, we very well may operate within the dramaturgical model; on the other hand, if we embrace the central metaphor that life is a jungle and "survival of the fittest" is the rule, then we may operate within the ethnomethodological model. Likewise, if we accept the central metaphor of "the Establishment," we may operate within the labeling model, or, if we subscribe, perhaps by default, to the central metaphor of fate, then we may operate within the existential model. (For a similar set of relationships, but based on linguistic models, see Lakoff and Johnson concerning "experiential gestalts" 77–86.)

The following schemata seek to highlight contrasts and similarities between the dramaturgical and labelling theory models of sociology, which are subtypes of symbolic interactionism, and the existential and ethnomethodological models of sociology, which are subtypes of phenomenology (St. Clair, "Language").

Dramaturgical Model

a. Social roles are created.
b. Individuals should perform in roles and use scripts.
c. Members are both audience and critic.
d. Stage fright can be enhanced.

Labelling Model

a. People share a common world of symbolism.
b. Members are taught views of the world.
c. Such teaching establishes norms.
d. These norms enable an insider/outsider distinction.

Existential Model

a. The world is without meaning.
b. Belief systems are arbitrary.

c. The world is full of alienation and insecurity.
   d. Conflict and negotiation are the norm.

Ethnomethodological

   a. Behavior is justified and excuses are explained.
   b. Face games are used to protect the member's identity.
   c. "Relationship games" involve "impression management."
   d. Members "struggle for the establishment of power."
   e. An inherent "right to control others" exists.
   f. Members have a need to re-affirm self-esteem.

Not only do central metaphors determine in large part our sociological models and how and what we view as coherent, but they also determine significant parts of our vocabulary. St. Clair argues that "language is never neutral" (*Social Metaphor* 41), and this lack of neutrality is proven when we examine our lexicon, for it can quickly indicate the operational central metaphor and sociological model. For example, if we are using the central metaphor of chance, we will likely include in our lexicon many of the following expressions:

> maybe I'll get lucky, good luck, chances are ... , the odds are against it, let's take a chance, let the chips fall where they may, Lady Luck smiled on me, the Man upstairs likes me, you pays your money and you takes your chances, he lucked out, he lucked up, it's not my day

Alternatively, someone who is using the central metaphor of machine might have a lexicon which includes the following expressions:

> he's wired too tight, learn the nuts and bolts of it, get cranked up, get in gear, stay in gear, can't get out of low gear, missed a gear, in high gear, hit the brakes, a little rusty, in sync, ginning right along

Clearly, our lexicon can indicate the central metaphor we are using.

Warrants

While we do not wear a lapel button announcing to the world which central metaphor we are employing or which epistemological framework we are operating within, both are indicated implicitly in a multitude of ways, such as through body language, lexicon, and prosodic features of spoken language.

From the beginning, this work has emphasized the explicit-implicit dynamic that involves the various elements of coherence. This part of the book examines an element of coherence that is a form of tacit knowledge and which is integral to the very notion of rhetoric. In classical rhetoric, this form of tacit knowledge was exemplified in the enthymeme, a truncated form of syllogism with one of the premises implied, and is, as Corbett puts it, "the instrument of deductive reasoning peculiar to the art of rhetoric" (74). But the minor or major premise of a syllogistic argument is not all that is implicit in the successful essay or composition.

When we compose an essay, we do not normally state our epistemological framework, nor the central metaphors we live by, although it is perfectly possible to do so. Likewise, we do not normally explain the sociological model we are operating within. Of course, we could inform our audience that we are strict empiricists who believe that life is best lived under the law of fang and claw (though this connection is not a necessary one), and that we role-play and engage in the manipulation of symbols, both linguistic and otherwise, in an effort to "come out on top" in this "civil" contest of life in which only the fittest survive. And of course, we might inform our audience of our epistemological framework, choice of central metaphors, and sociological model in a genuine effort to establish rapport, but normally, all of this and much more is implied when we produce an essay or composition, and this tacit knowledge, essential for successful communication between the writer and the reader, may be captured in a single concept: warrants.

In his *The Uses of Argument,* Stephen E. Toulmin argues against traditional symbolic logic as the truest form of argument. He raises the following questions, questions which bear directly on the notion of contextual salience:

> What things about the modes in which we assess arguments, the standards by reference to which we assess them and the manner in which we qualify our conclusions about them, are the same regardless of field (field-invariant),

and which of them vary as we move from arguments in one field to arguments in another (field-dependent)? How far, for instance, can one compare the standards of argument relevant in a court of law with those relevant to a mathematical proof or a prediction about the composition of a tennis team? (11)

What Toulmin is addressing here when he distinguishes between "field-invariant" and "field-dependent" is the notion of context, specifically, the notion of implied context or background knowledge which the writer can safely assume forms an implicit "bridge" between the writer and the audience. The "standards of argument" may well differ from a court of law to a mathematical proof to predictions of who will and who will not make the tennis team. The standards will vary because the context varies; indeed, even within argument types, e.g., within the field of law, the standards will vary, as tax lawyers learn very quickly when they seek to become trial lawyers. Thus, the notion of context is pivotal in the coherent argument, as it is in the coherent essay or composition.

Significantly, much of what is contextually salient in a rhetorical situation is implicit. In his model of argumentation, Toulmin calls the implicit part of the background information which forms an implicit bridge between the rhetor and the audience the warrant. It might also be thought of as the implicit and necessary part of a writer's register.

The concept of warrants in rhetoric entails many factors. When one considers writing in various disciplines, one notes that what is assumed for each discipline includes epistemological frame, arrangement, and lexicon. Writers of the scientific paper may be wed to empiricism for their epistemological frame. Also, they may follow a specified arrangement such as observations, hypothesis, hypothesis testing, results, and conclusions, as well as be expected to employ a lexicon specific to the field. Moreover, an "objective" tone will be assumed, and the use of passive voice will be acceptable and perhaps encouraged. In like manner, the writer of the literary essay will most likely operate unconstrained by empiricism, have much more freedom of arrangement, but also be expected to use a lexicon specific to literary criticism. The "subjective" tone may be quite acceptable, even encouraged for the interpretive portion of the paper, and passive voice will, in all likelihood, be discouraged.

Warrants, then, may vary from discipline to discipline, and when we write in specific disciplines, we must acquaint ourselves with the discipline's particular warrants and respect the bounds. If we use too much warrant, i.e., if we assume too much, we risk incoherence; if we use too little warrant, i.e., if we assume too little, we risk tedious repetition, much as if we were to avoid the use of pronouns and elect instead to name the proper noun at its every reference. In this latter case, warrants, in a sense, serve a shorthand function paralleling that of the pronoun in the linguistic perspective of coherence.

Moreover, and equally important, the appropriate warrant enables one physician to pick up a journal and read with confidence and efficiency an article written by another physician, or a biologist to read with confidence and efficiency an article written by another biologist, or a social worker to read with confidence and efficiency an article written by another social worker. Warrants are determined by a "match" at various levels of rhetoric: from a narrow match for writing done within particular disciplines by members of the discipline for members of the discipline, to a broad match when one writes for members of what Perelman and Olbrechts-Tyteca call the "universal audience" (30–35). Once the warrant is established, then such rhetorical features as arrangement, lexicon, and tone follow by mutual assent between writer and audience.

Contextually Salient Elements of Coherence

The contextually salient perspective of coherence is culturally related; thus, it often seems to be omnipresent and ubiquitous. However, it is often the most implicit aspect of coherence. The contextually salient perspective seldom manifests itself explicitly or directly through language meant to be understood at the literal level, as in the linguistic and cognitive perspectives, but rather in language meant to be understood at the interpretive level in the form of such key components of a composition as lexicon, grammatical structure (e.g., voice and nominalizations, etc.), rhetorical pattern of sentences (e.g., balanced, loose, or periodic), thesis placement, and prevalence of particular central cognitive processes (often resulting in emphasis on a particular arrangement or pattern of thought).

What follows is a summary listing of contextually salient elements of coherence. Just as the listing of the cognitive elements of coherence was not meant to be exhaustive, neither is this list meant to be exhaustive. Rather, it is offered in an attempt to draw appropriate attention to largely implicit elements of a text which traditionally have been overlooked or pointedly excluded with regard to coherence. We might recall that Halliday and Hasan seem to give equal status to both register and cohesion, yet the latter is the focus in *Cohesion in English*.

Indeed, according to Halliday and Hasan, "texture" (global coherence) is achieved through the mutually complementary relationship of "register" and "cohesion" (23). As noted above, the concept of warrants and all it entails may be regarded as the implicit and necessary part of a writer's register.

Halliday and Hasan define register as "the set of meanings, the configuration of semantic patterns, that are typically drawn upon under the specified conditions, along with the words and structures that are used in the realization of the meanings" (23). Halliday and Hasan thus acknowledge the essential nature of extra-textual elements in order for a text to evince coherence, but they limit their work to the surface language of a text, deliberately and explicitly excluding register, and thus warrants, from their study of cohesion in English.

Gutwinski goes even further with regard to extra-textual elements of cohesion. As noted in chapter two, he believes coherence to be unanalyzable in the linguistic sense because it deals with phenomena which "cannot be treated on a single level of analysis and some which are not open to linguistic analysis at all" (26). Such a position, which allows only for empirical data, bespeaks the epistemological framework *Naturwissenschaften* (natural sciences), and is an exclusionary one which does not begin to address the complex and multi-layered elements which function to cohere an essay or composition.

The following list, then, is an attempt to account for at least some of the major elements of coherence in the contextually salient perspective;

these elements, though implicit, are nonetheless essential. Indeed, they may be the most pervasive and powerful of all the elements of coherence, for they deal not only with epistemological frameworks, but also with one's values and belief systems.

Examples of Epistemological Frames

Geisteswissenschaften (the humanities): inclusive use of intangible and tangible data

Naturwissenschaften (the natural sciences): exclusive use of only tangible data

Examples of Central Metaphors

Cosmos: the metaphor which emphasizes the harmony, order, and balance in the universe

Growth: the metaphor which views the good as expansion or increasing consumption

Jungle: the metaphor which views life as the survival of the fittest

Chance: the metaphor which emphasizes the randomness and unpredictability of life

Fate: the metaphor which views life's events as foreordained

Journey: the metaphor which likens life to a trip: beginning, interim passage(s), and destination

The Establishment: the metaphor which acknowledges a controling status quo

Money: the metaphor that life has a cash nexus and everything is viewed in relation to this nexus

Machine: the metaphor that life is mechanistic, and accordingly is analyzable and predictable

Stage: the metaphor that life is drama and requires various roles to be played

Examples of Sociological Models

dramaturgical
labelling
phenomenological
ethnomethodological

Examples of Features Which Enable Warrants

lexicon
grammatical structure
arrangement
thesis placement
prevalence of particular central cognitive processes
rhetorical pattern of sentences
tone

An Explicit-Implicit Continuum

Our treatment of the **linguistic** perspective of coherence resulted in the continuum below:

<------EXPLICIT------------------------------------IMPLICIT----->

repetition
anaphora
cataphora
ellipsis   ellipsis

Because of the mandatory explicitness of the linguistic elements of coherence, all four categories—repetition, anaphora, cataphora, and ellipsis—are located at the explicit end of the continuum, but because ellipsis has an implicit component, it is also located at the implicit end of the continuum.

Unlike the linguistic elements of coherence, which always have a mandatory, explicit component manifested in the text through and by language expressly for co-referential purposes, the cognitive elements of coherence are often manifested in a liminal manner and serve as a threshold at which the explicit-implicit distinction blurs.

Consequently, the explicit-implicit continuum, with elements coded from both the **linguistic** and *cognitive* perspectives of coherence, approximates the following:

```
<-------EXPLICIT-------------limen---------------IMPLICIT------>
given/new relationship
                                          good continuation
                                          closure
                                          restructuring
                          central
                          cognitive
                          processes
repetition
anaphora
cataphora
ellipsis                                  ellipsis
```

Now, it is necessary to locate the elements of the contextually salient perspective of coherence on the explicit-implicit continuum.

The overwhelming use of language is not empirical reference, i.e., reference exclusively to the empirical here-and-now; rather, most language use is modal reference, i.e., reference to all situations and circumstances not in the empirical here-and-now. Just as the referents of this modal use of language are not located in the here-and-now, the contextually salient elements of coherence are not located within the text.

Consequently, the explicit-implicit continuum, with elements coded from the **linguistic**, *cognitive*, and *contextually salient* perspectives of coherence, approximates the following:

```
<-------EXPLICIT-------------limen---------------IMPLICIT------>
      given/new relationship                good continuation
                                            closure
                                            restructuring

                                            epistemological frames
                                            central metaphors
                                            sociological models
                                            warrants
                         central
                         cognitive
                         processes
  repetition
  anaphora
  cataphora
  ellipsis                                  ellipsis
```

This schema is far from complete, but it offers a set of elements from three different perspectives that may serve as a manageable framework within which we can better analyze and teach coherence. The schema suggests a complex and multi-layered continuum of elements which function to enable coherence. While this continuum reflects an explicit-implicit dynamic, it does not represent a configuration which integrates the three perspectives and their respective elements. In the next, and concluding, chapter of this work, such a configuration is offered.

CHAPTER FIVE

SYZYGY

This work on coherence began with an observation from Edward P. J. Corbett that coherence is a veritable morass. This may be so, but the following two passages from classical rhetoric's *On the Sublime* indicate that Longinus was not averse to struggling with this morass, for he wrote "... we see skill in invention, and due order and arrangement of matter, emerging as the hard-won result not of one thing nor of two, but of the whole texture of the composition" (43). He continued:

> Now, there inhere in all things by nature certain constituents which are part and parcel of their substance. It must needs be, therefore, that we shall find one source of the sublime in the systematic selection of the most important elements, and the power of forming, by their mutual combination, what may be called one body. (69)

I have sought to identify these "most important elements" so that teachers of rhetoric and composition, and particularly their students, will have a better idea of what a coherent text or communication entails. Perhaps more importantly, teachers and students may also have a better idea about why a particular text or communication fails to cohere and how to remedy the lack of coherence.

Toward this end, this work explores three lines of inquiry: a linguistic perspective, a cognitive perspective, and a contextually salient perspective. The linguistic elements serve a co-reference function, constitute sets with a relatively small number of words in a given text, occur frequently, and have a mandatory explicitness in which they represent the given in the given/new relationship and thus enable logical identity and consistency of reference.

The cognitive elements consist of the umbrella concepts of the given/new relationship, Gestalt, and central cognitive processes.

The contextually salient elements consist of epistemological frames, central metaphors, sociological models, and warrants as they serve to enable the coherence of an essay or composition. Much of the function of these elements is extra-textual and implicit, and much of the language used to signify them is at the interpretive level. These elements are pervasive and ubiquitous. In the implicit-explicit continuum below, the *contextually salient* elements are in *italics*, the **linguistic** elements are in **bold**, and ***cognitive*** elements are in ***bold italics***.

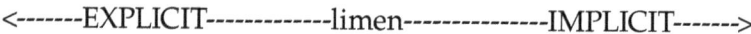

<-------EXPLICIT-------------limen---------------IMPLICIT------>

given/new relationship   ***good continuation***
                                            closure
                                            restructuring

                                            epistemological frames
                                            central metaphors
                                            sociological models
                                            warrants

                    central
                    cognitive
                    processes

repetition
anaphora
cataphora
ellipsis   **ellipsis**

The elements listed above are not intended to be inclusive; rather, they are meant to break new ground in coherence theory and to redistribute the burden of coherence from the sentence level and from the surface language of the text to a more inclusive and realistic tri-partite focus. In this sense, then, they may be thought of as the "certain constituents" to which Longinus refers when he writes "… there inhere in all things by nature certain constituents which are part and parcel of their substance" (69).

All three sets of elements—**linguistic**, *cognitive*, and *contextually salient*—interrelate in distinctive ways to achieve textual coherence. The linguistic elements create an explicit and consistent thread of co-reference, thus ensuring "the most fundamental principle of language: the normative principle of logical identity" (Waldron 197). This set of cohering elements performs the crucial role of maintaining the integrity of the nucleus of natural language logic, a nucleus which consists of logical identity and co-reference.

The cognitive elements encompass this nucleus of logical identity and co-reference and enable the generation and organization of content around and about it. These elements cross all registers and semantic domains and are universal for all humans. Significantly, the central cognitive processes are located at the limen of explicitness-implicitness, and their life on the boundary allows them to shift from the explicit to the implicit as linguistic convention or concerns of contextual salience dictate.

The contextually salient elements encompass the cognitive elements as well as the linguistic elements and establish the expectations and constraints of the rhetorical situation. These elements are not only the most implicit, but also the most pervasive, the most ubiquitous, and the most circumscribing.

Visual Metaphor of Coherence

The visual metaphor on the following page offers another way of viewing the elements of coherence and their interrelationships.

A Visual Metaphor of Coherence

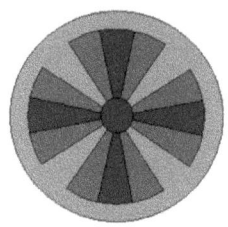

Elements   **Properties**

                    Linguistic Perspective

repetition   most explicit
anaphora   enables reference, co-reference, & logical identity,
cataphora   and thus
ellipsis   *comprises the nucleus of natural language logic*

                    Cognitive Perspective

given/new relationship   at explicit-implicit limen
good continuation   crosses all domains and registers
closure   universal for all humans and so
restructuring   *enables both invention and arrangement*
central cognitive processes

                    Contextually Salient Perspective

epistemological frames   most implicit
central metaphors   most circumscribing
sociological models   most pervasive and thus
warrants   *determines expectations & constraints of the rhetorical situation*
ellipsis

No metaphor is completely descriptive. The metaphor offered above, adapted from Niels Bohr's model of the atom, does not capture the pervasiveness of contextual salience. In order for it to do so, the model would have to be three dimensional with fibers or force fields of a constraining nature extending from it and throughout the three "levels." Nonetheless, this metaphor captures several vital aspects of the perspectives.

For instance, the overarching nature of contextual salience is accurately represented, as is the nucleus of natural language logic, the integrity of which is maintained by the linguistic level. Too, the visual metaphor places the cognitive level, whose central cognitive processes are liminal regarding explicit and implicit properties, between the most explicit level, the linguistic level, and the most implicit level, the contextual salience level.

Significantly, the three "concentric" levels of the visual metaphor comprise a continuum of more-or-less discrete "coherence fields" potentially in contact with any other "coherence field" on any level, thus simulating the property of parallel distributed processing.

Finally, instead of confining the focus of coherence to the surface of a text at sentence level, this visual metaphor enables one to comprehend better the multi-layered complexity inherent in coherent texts or communications.

Points of Departure for Teachers of Rhetoric and Composition

In "What Makes a Text Coherent?", Betty Bamberg tells us that "Our goal as writing teachers must be to create a classroom setting that enables students to understand what makes a text coherent" (427). Although *Beyond Cohesion: Toward a Theory of Coherence* is a book of theory for those working in rhetoric and composition, its theory and the components of its theory may serve as points of departure for pedagogy. To that end, I list the following, which, while not inclusive, may serve as guides or suggestions.

Parts to Whole and Whole to Parts

Coherence is defined as the comprehensive, systematic connection of constitutive elements of a text of logical discourse, with a consistent emphasis on the totality of the text and on the interrelatedness of its constituents (chapter one). Two significant notions are couched in this definition: the notion of parts, i.e., the "constituents," and the notion of whole, i.e., the "totality of the text." The parts to whole and whole to parts relationships are depicted in both the explicit-implicit continuum and the visual metaphor. The former offers constitutive elements along an explicit-implicit continuum; these constitutive elements comprise a totality resulting in the coherence of an essay or composition. Similarly, the visual metaphor offers a totality of constitutive elements in the form of the perspectives—the linguistic, cognitive, and contextually salient perspectives. In both the explicit-implicit continuum and the visual metaphor, as well as in the definition of coherence, the parts to whole and whole to parts relationships evince themselves as integral to an understanding of coherence. It follows, then, that an acute awareness of this relationship ought to be central to pedagogy.

Bottom Up and Top Down Processing

Any approach toward coherence that focuses on one particular language level, as in the *Harbrace College Handbook* with its focus on the sentence level, or on one discourse level, as in McCrimmon's *Writing with a Purpose* with its focus on the paragraph, falls short of the mark. Instead, one needs an approach which emphasizes the parts to whole and the whole to parts relationships.

As Bamberg tells us in "What Makes a Text Coherent?", "readers draw on their tacit knowledge at the level of the sentence and of the whole discourse by using a 'top-down,' 'bottom-up' strategy. That is, as they process individual words and sentences at the beginning of a text, they attempt to form an overall conception of the structure and meaning of the whole text into which they can fit the information that follows" (420).

If the teacher facilitates bottom up processing of elements in conjunction with top down processing, i.e., if the student is encouraged to see "the big picture" of the assignment, of what sort of text or communication might result, while also being encouraged to see how the elements may combine to cohere a text, then that student's prospects are enhanced. Hence, the writer would be actively engaged in dual tasks. An approach incorporating the parts to whole/whole to parts dynamic also meshes with studies in learning theory which suggest that we as individuals have different cognitive styles. Some of us tend to begin with "the big picture" and then "flesh it out," while others begin with several small observations and details and then build upon them until a coherent text emerges.

Ensuring the Implied Elements of Cultural Salience Are for the Good

The culturally salient elements enabling coherence are usually extra-textual or implied: warrants, central metaphors, sociological models, and epistemological frames. These implied elements can be used for good or ill. One way for teachers to ensure that they are used for good is through an optimal classroom ecology.

Asao Inoue offers a heuristic that can help teachers ensure that culturally salient elements, implied or overt, are used for socially just and intellectually healthy purposes. The parts of this heuristic ecology in the writing classroom are purposes, e.g., student placement or to get a grade (284); processes, e.g., designing, responding to, or evaluating a prompt (285); places, figurative or real (286–287); parts, e.g., codes, artifacts, or documents (287–288); power, e.g., as evinced in portfolio design or classroom proxemics (288–289); people, who are diverse racially and culturally (289–290); and products, either direct or indirect (290–291). Moreover, such an ecology in the classroom can help enable students to choose when and if to code switch, when and if to "code mesh," (Young et al., 2014, 66–86) and to work toward "a global citizenship ... [that] allows every student, regardless of their journeys, to be seen as a whole, legitimate person with rich language and literacy practices" (Alvarez and Wan, 216).

Linear and Non-Linear Aspects

If the cognitive perspective, and particularly if the contextually salient perspective, is accepted, then a pedagogical implication concerning linearity emerges: many of the cohering elements of successful composing are not linear (e.g., central cognitive processes, central metaphors, and warrants). In "Untold Stories," Sakeena Everett argues that teachers can show how "metaphors organize creatively, here cognitively, linguistically, and philosophically what we believe to be possible" (39). Everett shows how a student created and used the metaphor of a yellow school bus shackled with handcuffs (45) to move the student from the "banking metaphor" (49) of education to the bridging metaphor.

Teachers can engage students in non-linear thought such as that of a metaphor and then face the larger challenge of coaching and coaxing student writers into articulating their non-linear thought into linear language appropriate for the rhetorical context.

The Dual Nature of Central Cognitive Processes

Traditionally, words such as **however**, **although**, and **therefore** have been viewed as conjunctive adverbs or subordinate conjunctions, depending on whether they relate main clauses or subordinate clauses. From a purely grammatical or surface language view, this may be acceptable, but this position overlooks the dual nature of such transition words.

These words not only bridge, but actually are channels or kinds of thought. Central cognitive processes not only enable us to generate thoughts, but also to organize them.

Because of this dual nature, they are arguably the best examples of the fluid relationship between invention and arrangement and thus merit special emphasis.

Syzygy

As far as is known, no other beings in the cosmos have developed the scope and degree of spoken ability that we humans have, yet as wonderful as speech is, it alone would not have taken us very far from the cave. Written language, however, with its ability to hypostasize thought, thus enabling permanent records, reflection, and extended discourse capable of revision, exposes humans to seemingly infinite frontiers within the psyche and outside it, to the far, unfathomable reaches of space. Surely, then, to fashion coherent, extended, written discourse for a specific purpose to a specific audience regarding a specific occasion is to participate in a uniquely human endeavor.

In the discipline of astronomy, one learns of a phenomenon called syzygy. Syzygy is a natural alignment of elements—three celestial bodies—but it is not a continuous alignment, and it occurs only when certain conditions and perspectives coalesce; similarly, one may envision a kind of syzygy in the coalescing of conditions and perspectives when the writer successfully aligns the "certain constituents" of the three perspectives which are "part and parcel" of a coherent essay or composition: the linguistic, cognitive, and culturally salient perspectives. These constituents are myriad, intricate, and amazingly interwoven, yet if student writers can learn how to align these perspectives and coalesce their elements, then they may well experience a sense of the sublime which Longinus extolls. It is my hope that this book will help teachers of rhetoric and composition guide their students so that they may experience this sense of the sublime.

Appendix

This appendix serves two purposes:

1. Because I offer in *Beyond Cohesion: Toward a Theory of Coherence* an argument that, in essence, reduces a significant portion of Halliday and Hasan's *Cohesion in English* to a small number of elements which contribute fundamentally to the theory of coherence, and because I do not want to seem peremptory in this reduction, I offer the detailed argument below. I have the utmost respect for Halliday and Hasan and do not want to be viewed as sweeping past their work.
2. The appendix comprises a detailed linguistic argument which some readers may find worth their while.

Numbered headings are keyed to references in the body of the book. Italicized portions indicate especial relation to references in the body of the book.

(Unless otherwise indicated, all page numbers are from the edition of Halliday and Hasan's *Cohesion in English* as entered in the Works Cited of this book.)

****

A1. Register

Register is "the set of meanings, the configuration of semantic patterns, that are typically drawn upon under the specified conditions, along with the words and structures that are used in the realization of the meanings" (23). Here, too, we see Halliday and Hasan tend toward coherence as they thus acknowledge the essential nature of extra-textual elements in order for a text to evince coherence ("textuality"), but *they limit their work to the surface language of a text, deliberately and explicitly excluding register from their study of cohesion in English.* Nonetheless, their work concerning the cohesive elements of a text's surface language forms an important and substantial part of the linguistic perspective of coherence.

A2. Cohesion

For Halliday and Hasan, cohesion has two central and distinguishing properties. First, it is a relational system in which "one item provides the source for the interpretation of another" and as such is "the set of possibilities that exist in the language for making [a] text hang together: the potential that the speaker or writer has at his disposal" (18–19). Second, cohesion is also "a process, in the sense that it is the instantiation of this relation [between two items] in a text" and "always involves one item pointing to another" (18–19).

A3. Reference and Co-reference

A distinction needs to be made at this point, one concerning Halliday and Hasan's meaning of the word **reference**. Reference and logical identity form the nucleus of natural-language logic. Reference is the most fundamental property of language, the simple but absolutely essential characteristic enabling the link between linguistic symbol and the thing referred to. However, this fundamental meaning of reference is not what is meant by Halliday and Hasan. Rather, they use the word **reference** to mean co-reference, i.e., two or more words having the same referent. In this book, the word **reference** carries its fundamental meaning, and the word **co-reference** is used wherever Halliday and Hasan have used the word **reference**.

A4. The Tie as the Fundamental Cohesive Property

Central to Halliday and Hasan's approach to textual analysis is the notion of the tie, which they define as "a single instance of cohesion, a term for one occurrence of a pair of cohesively related items" (5). An example is "the relation between **them** and **six cooking apples**" in the following:

> [2:1] Wash and core six cooking apples. Put them into a fireproof dish.

A5. Immediate, Mediated, and Remote Ties

A tie, then, is "best interpreted as a RELATION between ... two elements," one of which presupposes the other; a tie is "also DIRECTIONAL," in that it is anaphoric ("presupposed element preceding") or cataphoric ("presupposed element following") (329). Ties may be "IMMEDIATE," "MEDIATED," or "REMOTE" as the following passage illustrates:

> [2:2] The last word ended in a long bleat, so like a sheep that Alice quite started (I). She looked at the Queen, who seemed to have suddenly wrapped herself up in wool (2). Alice rubbed her eyes, and looked again (3). She couldn't make out what had happened at all (4). Was she in a shop (5)? And was that really—was it really a **sheep** that was sitting on the other side of the counter (6)? Rub as she would, she could make nothing more of it (7). (qtd. in Halliday & Hasan 330)

Because the **she** in sentence (2) refers to **Alice** in sentence (1), and the two sentences are contiguous, the tie is immediate. If the ties occur in three or more contiguous sentences, then the ties are "MEDIATED," as for the **she** in (5) and **Alice** in (3); the **she** in (4) mediates because it, too, like the **she** in (5), presupposes **Alice** in (3). If a tie exists across a number of sentences with no mediated ties in the intervening sentences, then the tie is "REMOTE," as for **Rub as she would** in (7) and **Alice rubbed her eyes** in (3). In order for us to make sense of **Rub as she would**, we have to refer across prior, intervening, and non-mediating sentences to **Alice rubbed her eyes** in (3) (Halliday & Hasan 330–331).

Cohesive ties are of five types, reflecting the five sub-categories of cohesion: co-reference, substitution, ellipsis, conjunction, and lexical cohesion (4).

A6. The Cohesive Tie of Co-Reference

Halliday and Hasan treat the cohesive tie of co-reference as a "semantic," not a "grammatical," relation and view it as prior to the other types of cohesive ties. Co-reference is viewed directionally and semantically. Co-reference viewed directionally is of two broad categories: exophoric and endophoric.

A7. Exophoric Co-Reference

Exophoric co-reference deals with co-reference outside the text, i.e., to elements of the register, and thus is considered "situational" co-reference. Halliday and Hasan, drawing from Bernstein, illustrate exophoric co-reference with the following example:

> [2:3a] They're playing football and he kicks it and it goes through there it breaks the window and they're looking at it and he comes out and shouts at them because they've broken it so they run away and then she looks out and she tells them off. (qtd. in Halliday & Hasan 35)

In order for this passage to "make sense," we must have information concerning the referents of the pronouns, i.e., who they are, and perhaps what their roles are in the context of the passage (35). *Significantly for rhetoricians, Halliday and Hasan exclude exophoric reference from their study of cohesion in English.* The following paragraph offers a more extreme example:

[2:3b] They're playing and he kicks it and it goes through there it breaks the window and they're looking at it and they come out and shout at them because they've broken it so they run away and then she looks out and she tells them off.

A8. Endophoric Co-reference (anaphoric vs. cataphoric)

Endophoric co-reference deals with co-reference between items in a text and is considered "textual" co-reference. *Endophoric co-reference is the co-reference of primary concern for Halliday and Hasan. Endophoric co-reference subdivides into anaphoric and cataphoric co-reference, with anaphoric referring to an element located earlier in the text and cataphoric referring forward to an element in the text, as the following examples indicate*:

[2:4] anaphoric co-reference
Jon swims very well; **he** swam the English Channel.

[2:5] cataphoric co-reference
What I am going to say will interest you immensely.
Susan has decided to study medicine in Tibet.

A9. Personal, Demonstrative, and Comparative Co-reference

Co-reference viewed semantically is of three types: personal, demonstrative, and comparative. Personal co-reference is "by means of function in the speech situation" (37) and is exemplified in the following sentences:

[2:6] **I** bought a new car yesterday. (pronoun)
(We can also argue that **I** is substituting for a proper noun which lies outside the text, is therefore exophoric (cf. [2:3], not endophoric, and if we were to follow Halliday and Hasan's logic, the use of **I** would then not be textual. However, coherence as defined for this work encompasses exophoric co-reference. Regardless of the directionality, it is argued here that the use of **I** in this sentence is an example of substitution.)

[2:7] The salesman gave **me** a good deal. (pronoun)
  (Again, the pronoun **me** substitutes for a proper noun.)
[2:8] Now the car is **mine**. (determiner)
  (Here, **mine** substitutes for the noun phrase **my car**.)
[2:9] Now **my** bank account is nearly empty. (determiner)
  (For this last sentence, we can argue that **my** functions as a modifier in a noun phrase, not as a co-referent. Thus far, the uses of Halliday and Hasan's semantic co-reference are primarily that of substitution.)

Halliday and Hasan's second type of co-reference, demonstrative co-reference, is "essentially a form of verbal pointing" (deixis) according to proximity (57), and is realized

in words such as **this/these**, **here** (near), **that/those**, **there** (far), and the definite article **the**.

(Halliday and Hasan maintain that **the** should be included with the deictic words because **the** is a reduced form of **that**, and **the**, while making its referent definite, may refer to something in the register—exophorically—and thus qualifies as cohesive. It should be noted, however, that the focus of Halliday and Hasan throughout their book is on endophoric co-reference; thus, inclusion of **the** at the same status as the other deictic words because of an exophoric property is arguable.)

Examples of demonstrative co-reference are the following:

[2:10] I like the lions, and I like the polar bears. **These** are my favorites (60).
[2:11] We're going to the opera tonight. **This**'ll be our first outing for months (60).
  (We can argue that in [2:10], **These** is either a truncated or elliptical construction substituting for the noun phrase **these animals**, and that in [2:11], **This** substitutes for the noun phrase **our going**.)

Halliday and Hasan state that what "probably accounts for the majority of all instances" of demonstrative co-reference is extended co-reference, in which the demonstrative refers to a process or situation:

[2:12] They broke a Chinese vase.
  That was very careless. (66)
  That refers to the process involved which resulted in the breaking of the vases. (We can argue that **That** is actually another example of substitution: **That** = the breaking of the vase.)

Halliday and Hasan's third type of co-reference, comparative co-reference, is of two kinds, general and particular. General comparative co-reference is based on the notions that "likeness is a referential property," and a "thing cannot just be 'like'; it must be 'like something'" (18). The comparison "may be in the situation or in the text," it may be anaphoric and cataphoric, and it may be structural or non-structural, and if it is non-structural and in the text, then it is cohesive (78). (I argue in chapter three that the latitude of situations and conditions under which comparison operates, along with other reasons, makes it a central cognitive process and is not a form of co-reference.)

Examples of anaphoric and cataphoric general comparative co-reference are, respectively, the following:

> [2:13] Sam is at the door; I was expecting someone **different**.
> (We can argue that **different** is a truncated or elliptical form of the phrase **different than Sam**, and, in turn, that this phrase is a truncated form of the underlying clause **a person who differs from Sam**, which modifies **someone**. Thus, **different** is not used as co-reference, but is used to indicate comparison, which is treated in the cognitive perspective of coherence.)
> [2:14] She's a **different** breed **than** the one we had before.
> (Here, we can again argue that **different than** is not used as co-reference, but is used to indicate comparison, which is treated as a central cognitive process in the cognitive perspective in chapter three of this book.)

Additionally, Halliday and Hasan tell us, "the comparison may be internal—the likeness expressed as mutual likeness without a referent appearing as a distinct entity" (78), as the following illustrates:

> [2:15] Most people have the same breakfast every day. (meaning 'the same as every other day') (80)
> [2:16] The candidates gave three similar answers. (meaning 'similar to each other') (80)
> [2:17] All parties showed an identical reaction to the news.
> (meaning 'reacted in the same way as each other') (80)
> (In each of these cases, we can argue that the words **the same as**, **similar**, and **identical** principally indicate comparison, a central cognitive process, and not co-reference, i.e., none of the expressions share referents, but they indicate referents which share commonalities.)

Particular comparative co-reference "expresses comparability between things in respect of a particular property.

> [2:18] We don't need any **more** mistakes. [2:19] The hare ran fast**er**.
> [2:20] The sun shines bright**er**.
>> (We can make two additional arguments here: 1) each of these examples has elliptical constructions, e.g., [2:18] "We don't need any more mistakes (than we already have)" or [2:19] "The hare ran faster (than the tortoise) "; 2) comparison, not co-reference, is indicated by comparative forms **more** and **-er**.)

Curiously, Halliday and Hasan end their discussion of co-reference with the statement that "the different forms of cohesion are nowhere sharply set apart one from another" (87).

A10. Two Fundamental Observations Regarding Co-reference

In sum, from the examples above, we can make two observations. *First, much of co-reference can be seen as a form of substitution. Second, those examples of co*-reference which are not substitution can be seen as forms of comparison, a central cognitive process. Such recategorization simplifies the linguistic perspective of coherence.

A11. The Cohesive Tie of Substitution

Halliday and Hasan's second sub-category of cohesion is substitution. Halliday and Hasan argue that substitution is a relation between linguistic items, such as words or phrases;

where co-reference is a relation between meanings … co-reference is a relation on the semantic level, whereas substitution is a relation on the … level of grammar and vocabulary.

(89) (They add that ellipsis "can be defined as substitution by zero … but the mechanisms involved in the two [substitution and ellipsis] are rather different, … and in the case of ellipsis, fairly complex" [88–89].)

Examples of co-reference are the following:

[2:21] John has moved to a new house. He had **it** built last year. (54)
[2:22] Who are those colourful characters?
    Those must be the presidential guards. (63)
[2:23] The little dog barked as noisily as the big **one**. (82)

Examples of substitution are the following:

[2:24] My axe is too blunt. I must get a sharper **one**. (89) [2:25] What kind of engines do you want?
    Ones with whistles, or **ones** without? (92)
[2:26] These grapefruit smell more bitter than the last **ones** we had. (109) (Halliday and Hasan argue that **ones** is an example of substitution if the grapefruit also taste more bitter, but if they taste the same, then **ones** is an example of co-reference, not substitution.)

Although Halliday and Hasan argue co-reference occurs at the "semantic level," and that substitution occurs at the level of "grammar" and "vocabulary," when we examine their examples, we find the distinction to be nebulous, for each of their co-reference examples, [2:21] and [2:22], and their substitution example, [2:25], indicate the same referent; and their co-reference example, [2:23], and each of their substitution examples, [2:24] and [2:26], indicate different referents. What we do find in common for all examples is that substitution of a pro-form occurs. Thus, if we omit the co-reference/substitution distinction (or the semantic/grammatical distinction), we can avoid altogether the sort of puzzling, "smell" vs. "taste" contretemps presented by the grapefruit example [2:25].

Substitution is of three types: nominal, verbal, and clausal. Nominal substitution uses the words **one, ones**, or **same**; verbal substitution uses the word **do**; and clausal substitution uses the words **so** or **not**. These word lists are virtually inclusive, with only a few exceptions: the expressions **do so**, and **do the same**, about which there is some "indeterminacy," and general words such as **thing**, "where substitution shades into lexical cohesion" (91).

Examples of nominal substitution are found in [2:24], [2:25], and [2:26] above.

Examples of verbal substitution are in the following sentences:

[2:27] … the words did not come the same as they used to **do**. (substitution for **come**) (112)

[2:28] I don't know the meaning of half those long words, and, what's more, I don't believe you **do** either!
(substitution for **know the meaning of half those long words**) (112)

Halliday and Hasan note that for **do** substitution, "the contrastive element which provides the context for the substitution is located within the same clause," as in [2:27] and [2:28] above, unlike in clausal substitution (below), in which "the clause is presupposed, and the contrasting element is outside the clause" (130).

Clausal substitution occurs in the environment of hypotaxis, i.e., one clause depends on another semantically, but not through structural embedding (136). Examples of clausal substitution are in the following sentences:

[2:29] Is there going to be an earthquake?
It says **so**. (**so** substitutes for the entire clause **there is going to be an earthquake**, with **says** serving as the contrastive environment) (130)
[2:30] (reported clause)
'… if you've seen them so often, of course you know what they're like.'
'I believe **so**,' Alice replied thoughtfully. (131)
[2:31] (conditional clause)
Everyone seems to think he's guilty. If **so**, no doubt he'll offer to resign. (134)
[2:32] (modalized clause)
'Oh, I beg your pardon!' cried Alice hastily, afraid that she had hurt the poor animal's feelings. 'I quite forgot you didn't like cats.'
'Not like cats!' cried the Mouse, in a shrill, passionate voice. 'Would you like cats if you were me?'
'Well, perhaps **not**,' said Alice in a soothing tone… . (134)

Lastly, regarding the use of **not**, Halliday and Hasan relate that "the negative form of the clausal substitute is **not**" (133), as in the following example:

[2:33] Has everyone gone home?   I hope not. (133)

Halliday and Hasan's treatment of substitution not only offers numerous examples illustrating how it enables cohesive ties in texts, but it also delineates kinds of substitution—nominal, verbal, and clausal, and in their contrast of verbal and clausal substitution, they draw attention to the hypotactic environment, an environment which accounts for inter-clausal cohesive ties.

A12. The Cohesive Tie of Ellipsis

Ellipsis is the third major sub-category of cohesion in Halliday and Hasan's schema, and although they state that "ellipsis is simply 'substitution by zero,'" they argue that for their purposes, it is "more helpful to treat the two [substitution and ellipsis] separately" because "they are two different kinds of structural mechanism, and hence show rather different patterns" (142). (It is interesting to note what may be some inconsistency on Halliday and Hasan's part in their using a structural property, i.e., "kinds of structural mechanism," to justify their treatment of ellipsis, while they continue to categorize ellipsis as "non-structural.")

Halliday and Hasan seem a bit uncertain as to how to justify their assigning ellipsis unto its own category, for in one sentence they write "we can take as a general guide the notion that ellipsis occurs when something that is structurally necessary is left unsaid," and in the very next sentence they state "that the essential characteristic of ellipsis is that something which is present in the selection of an underlying ('systemic') option is omitted in the structure—whether or not the resulting structure is in itself 'incomplete'" (144). Then, by way of summary, they state again that the difference between substitution and ellipsis is that in the former a substitution counter occurs in the slot, and this must therefore be deleted if the presupposed item is replaced, whereas in the latter the slot is empty—there has been substitution by zero. (145)

Halliday and Hasan do not offer examples to illustrate this difference; however, we might assume that the following sentences illustrate how "substitution counter occurs in the slot," and how it "must therefore be deleted if the presupposed item is replaced" (145):

[2:34] original: John is building a house.
[2:35] substitution: He is building a house.
    (**He** is the "substitution counter" and presupposes **John**.)

By replacing the presupposed item, **John**, with **Sue**, we have

[2:36] original: Sue is building a house.
[2:37] substitution: She is building a house.

Clearly, the substitution counter is not deleted, but merely replaced by another substitution counter. Consider an example with ellipsis, i.e., substitution by zero:

[2:38] original: One rabbit ran fast, and another rabbit ran slowly.
[2:39] substitution: One rabbit ran fast, and another **(zero)** ran slowly.

By replacing the presupposed item, **rabbit**, with **dog**, we have

[2:40] original: One dog ran fast, and another dog ran slowly.
[2:41] substitution: One dog ran fast, and another **(zero)** ran slowly.

Hence, the structural mechanisms involved are not of "two different kinds" (142) unless we assume the "substitution counters", i.e., the instantiated nominal, verbal, clause, or zero items, to differ in non-semantic ways; further, the very same structural mechanism occurs, viz., the structural operation of substitution of co-referential items. Moreover, the underlying semantic status, not surface representation, of the "presupposed item" and the "substitution counter" is the determining factor in this aspect of cohesion: their underlying semantic status must be that of co-reference, and it matters not whether the substitution counter is zero or an instantiated nominal, verbal, or clause. The structural operation which effects the substitution is identical, and co-reference of the presupposed item and the substitution item ensures comprehension.

    Halliday and Hasan also argue that much of the distinction between substitution and ellipsis rests on the notions of single-element omission and branching clauses. Halliday and Hasan hold that single-element omission does not occur "WHERE THAT ELEMENT IS OTHERWISE OBLIGATORY" (205), as in the following examples:

[2:42] Has she taken her medicine?
[2:43] She has taken.
   (in this unacceptable sentence, the single element, the complement, has been omitted) (202)

However, we should consider an example of theirs before accepting their argument. In the following two sentences, the second sentence omits a single element, the complement, but according to Halliday and Hasan, this is not ellipsis because it is not "an instance of omission, and involves no presuppositions of any kind" (204), but rather an example of a systematic variant "in which nothing is omitted, any more than an expression of time or place can be said to be 'omitted' from a clause which does not contain one" (204).

[2:44] Simon's playing.
[2:45] Let's not interrupt. (204)

First, it is arguable that something has been omitted on two counts. A feature of English is its tendency toward the pattern Subject-Verb-Object (or Complement); English is commonly referred to as an SVO language, and as such, native speakers of English usually deem a Subject-Verb sentence incomplete if the verb is used in a transitive sense. For example, most native speakers of English find incomplete the following utterance if no object has been previously identified:

[2:46] Let's watch. (or Let's not watch.) Likewise incomplete is,
[2:47] Let's interrupt. (or Let's not interrupt.)

Native speakers would feel something had been omitted in [2:46] and in [2:47]. Likewise, if native speakers are presented with the sentences

[2:48] Simon's playing.
[2:49] Let's not interrupt.

and then are asked "Let's not interrupt 'what?'" they will normally answer "Simon" or "Simon's playing."

Thus, it seems that an omission has occurred in the sentence "Let's not interrupt." Halliday and Hasan do not explain the term "systematic variant," but whatever it is, we cannot deny the native speaker's intuition that an omission has occurred in "Let's not interrupt." Although the native speaker might not categorize it as such, it is an omission of a single element. Moreover, such an omission is not the same as the "omission" of "time" or "place" from a sentence, since virtually all utterances assume the metaphysical constants of time and place. Indeed, that is why they are "unmarked" in dialog, and why speakers signify a specific, non-metaphysical meaning of time and place by using definite, explicit "markers" such as the words **here, now, there**, and **then** whenever such reference is necessary for coherence.

Much of the rest of the argument that ellipsis is something more than zero substitution and hence merits its own category lies with ellipsis in question-and-answers such as the following:

[2:50] Is it Tuesday?
[2:51] I don't know. (212)
[2:52] Can you make it stand up?
[2:53] If you keep still. (213)
[2:54] When did they cancel the booking?
[2:55] Did they? (213)
[2:56] John's coming to dinner.
[2:57] John? (215)
[2:58] John's coming to dinner.
[2:59] And Mary? (215)

In these cases, Halliday and Hasan do not contest the omission as they do in sentences such as

[2:60] Simon's playing.
[2:61] Let's not interrupt. (204)

Finally, and perhaps most telling for the composition teacher who deals with problems in ellipsis resulting from tangled clauses in student writing, Halliday and Hasan argue that ellipsis does not occur in the following "branched" clauses:

[2:62] Either Peter will play his cello, or Sally her guitar. (203)
[2:63] The cat catches mice in the summer.
    And the dog rabbits. (203)

[2:64] The cat won't catch mice in winter.
   Nor the dog rabbits. (203)
[2:65] Sybil takes coffee very strong, but Joan very weak. (203)

Halliday and Hasan disqualify these sentences from exhibiting ellipsis on two grounds: (1) ellipsis for them involves "a form of pre-supposition between sentences," not within a sentence (203); and (2) the omission deals with the omission of "single elements of clause structure (as well as structures of any other rank)," i.e., with structure, and "we [Halliday and Hasan] are confining our definition of ELLIPSIS to its non-structural, cohesive sense" (203).

Accordingly, Halliday and Hasan argue that [2:63] and [2:64] do not exhibit ellipsis because, in fact, they are actually one sentence.

[2:66] The cat catches mice in the summer.
   And the dog rabbits. (203)
[2:67] The cat won't catch mice in winter.
   Nor the dog rabbits. (203)

However, consider the following versions of Julius Caesar's famous triplet:

[2:68] I came to Gaul.
   I saw Gaul.
   I conquered Gaul.
[2:69] I came.
   I saw.
   I conquered.
[2:70] I came; I saw; I conquered.
[2:71] I came, I saw, I conquered.

Is [2:68] three sentences? Most composition teachers would probably respond yes. Does ellipsis occur in example [2:68]? Most composition teachers would probably respond no. Is [2:69] three sentences? Again, most teachers of English would respond yes. Does ellipsis occur in [2:69]? Most composition teachers would probably respond yes. Is [2:70] three sentences? Here most composition teachers might hesitate. Is the semicolon a weak period, making [2:70] three sentences, or is the semicolon a strong comma, making [2:70] a single sentence? According to Halliday and Hasan, if we view [2:70] as three sentences, then ellipsis occurs, but if we views [2:70] as a single sentence, then ellipsis does not occur. Is [2:71] three sentences? Most composition teachers would respond no, that [2:71] is a single sentence.

Does ellipsis occur in [2:71]? Most composition teachers would respond yes, ellipsis does occur. How can this be? Does ellipsis, a significant feature of cohesion, hinge on whether a string of clauses is separated by semi-colons, commas, or periods? Surely not, for the semantic relationships are the same in each of the examples. Moreover, Halliday and Hasan argue that sentences like those below do not exhibit ellipsis because in each case the omission deals with the omission of "single elements of clause structure (as well as structures of any other rank)," and "we [Halliday and Hasan] are confining our definition of ELLIPSIS to its non-structural, cohesive sense" (203):

[2:72] Either Peter will play his cello, or Sally her guitar. (203)
[2:73] Sybil takes coffee very strong, but Joan very weak. (203)

However, the position regarding the omission of a single element can be countered with Halliday and Hasan's own example below in which a single element has been omitted.

[2:44] Simon's playing.
[2:45] Let's not interrupt. (204)

This argument, as stated earlier, is based on the SVO (Complement) tendency in the English language. The native speaker intuits that something has been omitted in [2:45] and will easily supply a suitable element to "complete" the sentence. In addition, such an omission, contrary to Halliday and Hasan's position, is not the same as the "omission" of "time" or "place" from a sentence, but instead is an omission of a situation-specific element unique to that speech act.

Indeed, Wolfgang Dressler argues that "conditions triggering explicit and elliptic anaphoric transformations ... are often similar," so similar that he posits, citing various scholars (Lakoff, Green, Dougherty, & Steinitz) a universal condition for both explicit and implicit (elliptical) anaphoric transformations: "recoverability or possibility of substitution," and that this is "true for deletion and anaphoric pronouns such as 'he, she, it' or pseudo-pronominal nouns" (205).

A13. Ellipsis a Form of Substitution

In light of the above arguments, and in light of Halliday and Hasan's uncertainty over the status of ellipsis, *I will, for the purposes of this approach to coherence, consider ellipsis a form of substitution, and one which is achieved through a structural operation involving the substitution of a zero item co-referential with the presupposed item. (For additional arguments supporting this position, we can read Dressler, Lakoff, Green, Dougherty, and Steinitz.)*

A14. Cohesive Tie of Conjunction

Moreover, *conjunction is better examined in the cognitive perspective of coherence because conjunctions indicate not only the basic temporal-spatial relationships of thought, but also the complex logical structures of the central cognitive processes. Thus, conjunctions indicate underlying, fundamental, and complex cognitive processes.*

Further, as we will see in chapter three, conjunction is inextricably bound to structure, for it is the role of conjunctions to indicate not only the basic temporal-spatial relationships of thought, but also the complex logical structures of the central cognitive processes.

A15. The Tie of Lexical Cohesion

Lexical cohesion is, as Halliday and Hasan maintain, non-structural in the sense that the ties enabling lexical cohesion are "associative" in nature (De Saussure 123, 125–127); these associational ties relate to semantic domains, which are integral to the cognitive and contextually salient perspectives of coherence addressed later in this work. Lexical cohesion is, however, structural in the sense that the meanings represented by the vocabulary of any semantic domain are wed to forms which, although arbitrary as Ferdinand de Saussure noted, are forms nonetheless.

Thus, the structural vs. non-structural dichotomy is an unnecessary dichotomy, one founded on the assumption that form (structure) can be separated from meaning. Form and meaning can no more be separated than can language from the development of higher-order thought.

In sum, *lexical cohesion subdivides into two categories, natural and synthetic semantic domains, with natural domains better examined from the cognitive perspective because they are products of evolved cognitive processes, and synthetic domains better examined from the contextually salient perspective because they are determined by cultural forces.*

Works Cited

Alvarez, Sara P., and Amy J. Wan. "Global Citizenship as Literacy: A Critical Reflection for Teaching Multilingual Writers." *Journal of Adolescent & Adult Literacy*, vol. 63, no. 2, September/October 2019, 213–216.
Araszkiewicz, Michal, and Jaromir Savelka. *Coherence: Insights from Philosophy, Jurisprudence and Artificial Intelligence.* Basel, Switzerland: Springer, 2013.
Aristotle. *Aristotle's Theory of Poetry and Fine Art.* 4th ed. Trans. S. H. Butcher. New York: Dover, 1955.
Aristotle. *The Rhetoric of Aristotle.* Trans. Lane Cooper. Englewood Cliffs: Prentice-Hall, 1960.
Bain, Alexander. *English Composition and Rhetoric.* New York: Appleton, 1890.
Bamberg, Betty. "What Makes a Text Coherent?" *College Composition and Communication*, vol. 34, December 1983, pp. 417–429.
Baumgratz, T., M. Cramer, and M. B. Plenio. "Quantifying Coherence." *Physical Review Letters*, vol. 113, no. 14, 2014, p. 140401.
Beaugrande, Robert de. *Text Production: Toward a Science of Composition.* Norwood: Ablex, 1984.
Beaugrande, Robert de. *Text, Discourse, and Process: Toward a Multidisciplinary Science of Texts.* Norwood: Ablex, 1980.
Bever, Thomas, James Lackner, and Richard Kirk. "The Underlying Structures of Sentences are the Primary Units of Immediate Speech Perception." *Perception and Psychophysics*, vol. 5, 1969, pp. 225–234.
Bloomfield, Leonard. *Language.* New York: Holt, Rinehart, & Winston, 1933.

Bransford, John, and Jeffrey Franks. "Abstraction of Linguistic Ideas." *Cognitive Psychology*, vol. 2, 1971, pp. 331–350.

Bransford, John, Richard Barclay, and Jeffrey Franks. "Sentence Memory: A Constructive versus an Interpretive Approach." *Cognitive Psychology*, vol. 3, 1972, pp. 193–209.

Brown, Richard. A *Poetics for Sociology: Towards a Logic of Discovery for the Human Sciences.* Boston: Cambridge University Press, 1979.

Bruner, Jerome. *Studies in Cognitive Growth.* New York: John Wiley, 1966.

Campbell, Kim Sydow. *Coherence, Continuity, and Cohesion: Theoretical Foundations for Document Design.* London: Routledge, 1994.

Canagarajah, Suresh. "Weaving the Text: Changing Literacy Practices and Orientations." *College English*, vol. 82, no. 1, September 2019, pp. 7–28.

Carrell, Patricia L. "Cohesion Is Not Coherence." *TESOL Quarterly*, vol. 16, no. 4, December 1982, pp. 479–488.

Cawdrey, Robert. *A Table Alphabeticall of Hard English Words* (1604). Gainesville: Scholars' Facsimiles & Reprints, 1966.

cognition. *Webster's Seventh New Collegiate Dictionary.* Springfield, MA: G & C Merriam, 1965.

cognizance. *Webster's Seventh New Collegiate Dictionary.* Springfield, MA: G & C Merriam, 1965.

coherence. *The Compact Edition of the Oxford English Dictionary.* Oxford: Oxford University Press, 1971.

coherence. *Webster's Third International Dictionary.* Ed. P. Gove. Springfield: G & G Merriam, 1968.

Corbett, Edward. *Classical Rhetoric for the Modern Student.* New York: Oxford University Press, 1971.

Corder, Jim. Personal interview. Department of English, Texas Christian University. Fort Worth, Texas. September, 1985.

Corder, Jim, and John Ruszkiewicz. *Handbook of Current English.* Glenview IL: Scott, Foresman, 1985.

Davidson, Donald. *American Composition and Rhetoric.* New York: Scribner's, 1943.

Davies, Keith, and Yitzhak Spiegel. *Biological Control of Parasitic Nematodes: Building Coherence Between Microbial Ecology and Molecular Mechanisms.* London: Springer, 2011.

De Lange, William. *A Dictionary of Japanese Proverbs.* Warren, CT: Floating World Editions, 2013.

Dilthey, Wilhelm. *Essay of Philosophy.* Trans. Stephen Emery & William Emery. New York: AMS Press, 1985.

Dilthey, Wilhelm. *Introduction to the Human Sciences.* Ed. & Trans. Ramon Betanzos. Detroit: Wayne State University Press, 1988.

Dougherty, Ray C. "An Interpretive Theory of Pronominal Reference." *FoL*, vol. 5, 1969, pp. 488–519.

Dressler, Wolfgang U. "Towards a Semantic Deep Structure of Discourse Grammar." *Papers from the Sixth Regional Meeting of the Chicago Linguistics Society.* Chicago: University of Chicago Department of Linguistics, 1970.

Dressler, Wolfgang U. "Morphology." *Handbook of Discourse Analysis,* vol. 2. Ed. Teun A. van Dijk. London: Academic, 1985. 77–86.

Everett, Sakeena. "Untold Stories." *Research in the Teaching of English,* vol. 53, no. 1, August 2018, pp. 34–57.

Faigley, Lester. *The Penguin Handbook.* New York: Longman, 2006. Print.

Flower, Linda. "Writer-Based Prose: A Cognitive Basis for Problems in Writing." *College English,* vol. 41, 1979, pp. 19–37.

Fodor, Jerry. *The Modularity of Mind.* Cambridge, MA: MIT Press, 1983.

Fuller, Thomas. *The Appeal of Injured Innocence.* London: W. Godbid, 1659.

Glass, Arnold, Keith Holyoak, and John Santa. *Cognition.* Reading, MA: Addison-Wesley, 1979.

Gleason, H. A. *Linguistics and English Grammar.* New York: Holt, Rinehart, & Winston, 1965.

Gleitman, Henry. *Psychology.* New York: Norton, 1981.

Green, Georgia M. "On **Too** and **Either**, and Not Just **Too** and **Either** Either." *Papers from the 4th Regional Meeting.* Chicago Linguistic Society, 1968.

Gutwinski, Waldemar. *Cohesion in Literary Texts: A Study of Some Grammatical and Lexical Features of English Discourse.* The Hague: Mouton, 1976.

Hacker, Dianna, and Nancy Sommers. *The Bedford Handbook.* Boston: Bedford/St. Martin's, 2010. Print.

Hairston, Maxine, and John Ruszkiewicz. *The Scott, Foresman Handbook for Writers.* New York: HarperCollins, 1991.

Hall, Dennis. Personal Interview of Edward P. J. Corbett. Ohio State University. Columbus, Ohio. June, 1969.

Halliday, M. A. K., and R. Hasan. *Cohesion in English.* London: Longman, 1976.

Halliday, M. A. K., and R. Hasan. "Categories of the Theory of Grammar." *Word,* vol. 17, 1961, pp. 241–292.

Halliday, M. A. K., and R. Hasan. "Descriptive Linguistics in Literary Studies." *English Studies Today, Third Series.* Ed. G. I. Duthie. Edinburgh: University Press, 1962. 56–59.

Halliday, M. A. K., and R. Hasan. "The Linguistic Study of Literary Texts." *Proceedings of the Ninth International Congress of Linguists.* Ed. Horace G. Lunt. The Hague: Mouton, 1964. 302–307.

Halliday, M. A. K., and R. Hasan. "Linguistic Function and Literary Style: An Inquiry into the Language of William Golding's *The Inheritors.*" *Literary Style: A Symposium.* Ed. Seymour Chatman. London: Oxford University Press, 1971. 330–365.

Harris, Zellig. "Discourse Analysis." *Language,* vol. 28, 1952, pp. 1–30.

Hasan, Ruquaia. "A Linguistic Study of Contrasting Features in the Style of Two Contemporary English Prose Writers." Diss. University of Edinburgh, 1964.

Hasan, Ruquaia. "Linguistics and the Study of Literary Texts." *Etudes de Linguistique Appliquee*, vol. 5, 1967, pp. 106–121.

Hasan, Ruquaia. "Grammatical Cohesion in Spoken and Written English: Part One" (Paper No. 7) *Programme in Linguistics and English Teaching*. London: Longmans, 1968.

Hegel, G. *The Philosophy of History*. Trans. J. Bibree. New York: Dover, 1956.

Hillocks, George, Jr. *Research on Written Composition*. Urbana: ERIC/NCTE, 1986.

Hirsch, E. D., Jr. *Validity in Interpretation*. New Haven, CT: Yale University Press, 1967.

Hobbes, Thomas. *Decameron Physiologicum: Or, Ten Dialogues of Natural Philosophy*. W. Crook, 1608.

Hodges, John C., and Mary E. Whitten. *Harbrace College Handbook*. New York: HBJ, 1977.

Horace. "Art of Poetry." *Critical Theory Since Plato*. Ed. Hazard Adams. San Diego: HBJ, 1971. 68–75.

Inoue, Asao B. *Antiracist Writing Assessment Ecologies: Teaching and Assessing Writing for a Socially Just Future*. Fort Collins, Colorado: WAC Clearinghouse, 2015.

Jones, Roger. *Physics as Metaphor*. New York: Meridian, 1982.

Jung, Cart. *Aspects of the Feminine*. Trans. R. F. C. Hull. Princeton, NJ: Princeton University Press, 1982.

Kameda, N. *Business Communication Toward Transnationalism: The Significance of Cross Cultural Business English and Its Role*. Tokyo: Kindai Bungeisha, 1996.

Kaplan, Robert B. *The Anatomy of Rhetoric: Prolegomena to a Functional Theory of Rhetoric*. Philadelphia: Center for Curriculum Development, 1972.

Kaplan, Robert B. "Cultural Thought Patterns in Inter-Cultural Education." *Readings on English as a Second Language*. Ed. Kenneth Croft. Cambridge, MA: Winthrop, 1980. 399–418.

Kintsch, Walter, and Teun A. van Dijk. "Towards a Model of Text Comprehension and Production." *Psychological Review*, vol. 85, 1978, pp. 363–394.

Knoblauch, C. H., and Lil Brannon. *Rhetorical Traditions and the Teaching of Writing*. Upper Montclair, NJ: Boynton/Cook, 1984.

Kuhn, Thomas. *The Structure of Scientific Revolutions*. Chicago: University of Chicago Press, 1970.

Lakoff, George. "A Figure of Thought." *Metaphor and Symbolic Activity*, vol. 3, 1985–1986, pp. 215–225.

Lakoff, George. "Pronouns and Reference." *The Linguistics Club*. Bloomington, IN: Indiana University, 1968.

Lakoff, George, and Mark Johnson. *Metaphors We Live By*. Chicago: University of Chicago Press, 1980.

Lanham, Richard. *A Handlist of Rhetorical Terms*. Berkeley: University of California Press, 1969.

Lawrence, Mary. *Writing as a Thinking Process*. Ann Arbor, MI: University of Michigan Press, 1972.

Leach, Edmund. *Culture and Communication: The Logic by Which Symbols are Connected*. Cambridge, England: Cambridge University Press, 1976.

Lee, Jerry Won. *Locating Translingualism*. New York: Cambridge University Press, 2022.
Levelt, Willem. "A Survey of Studies in Sentence Perception: 1970–1976." *Studies in the Perception of Language*. Eds. Willem Levelt & Giovanni Flores d'Arcais. New York: Wiley, 1978, 1–74.
Lindemann, Erika, ed. *CCCC Bibliography of Composition & Rhetoric 1987*. Carbondale: Southern Illinois University Press, 1987.
Longinus. *Longinus on the Sublime*. Trans. W. R. Roberts. Cambridge, England: Cambridge University Press, 1935.
Markels, Robin B. "Cohesion Paradigms in Paragraphs." *College English*, vol. 45, 1983, pp. 450–464.
Markels, Robin B. *A New Perspective on Cohesion in Expository Paragraphs*. Carbondale: Southern Illinois University Press, 1984.
Maurer, David W. *Whiz Mob*. New Haven: College & University Press, 1964.
metaphor. *The American Heritage Dictionary of the English Language*. Boston: Houghton Mifflin, 1978.
Minsky, Marvin. "A Framework for Representing Knowledge." *The Psychology of Computer Vision*. Ed. P. Winston. New York: McGraw, 1975.
MLA International Bibliography/ebsco host. web 13 Sep 2022.
Montaño-Harmon, María Rosario. "Discourse Features of Written Mexican Spanish: Current Research in Contrastive Rhetoric and Its Implications." *Hispania*, vol. 74, no. 2, May, 1991. pp. 417–425.
Murray, Donald. *A Writer Teaches Writing*. New York: Holt, Rinehart, & Winston, 1968.
Noble Banadda. Next Einstein Forum. NEF Fellow. nef.org/fellow/noble-banadda/. web 2022.
Ohmann, Richard. "In Lieu of a New Rhetoric." *College English*, vol. 26, 1964a, pp. 17–22.
Ohmann, Richard. "Generative Grammars and the Concept of Literary Style." *Word*, vol. 20, 1964b, pp. 423–439.
Perelman, C., and L. Olbrechts-Tyteca. *The New Rhetoric*. Trans. John Wilkinson and Purcell Weaver. Notre Dame, IN: University of Notre Dame Press, 1971.
Piaget, Jean. *Judgment and Reasoning in the Child*. New York: Harcourt, Brace, 1928.
Qin, Cailing. "The Impact of Cultural Thought Patterns Upon English Writing." *Cross-Cultural Communication*, vol. 13, no. 10, 2017, pp. 10–13.
Quine, W. V. O. "Two Dogmas of Empiricism." *Necessary Truth*. Ed. R. C. Sleigh. Englewood Cliffs, NJ: Prentice-Hall, 1972.
Quirk, Randolph, Sidney Greenbaum, Geoffrey Leech, and Jan Svartvik. *A Grammar of Contemporary English*. London: Longman, 1972.
Richards, I. A. *The Philosophy of Rhetoric*. New York: Oxford University Press, 1936.
Rommetveit, R. *On Message Structure: A Framework for the Study of Language and Communication*. New York: Wiley, 1974.
Saussure, Ferdinand de. *Course in General Linguistics*. Trans. Wade Baskin. New York: Philosophical Library, 1959.
Schank, Roger C., and Robert P. Abelson. *Scripts, Plans, Goals, and Understanding*. New York: Wiley, 1974.

Seddon, Fred. "Rand and Rescher on Truth." *Journal of Ayn Rand Studies,* vol. 8, no. 1, 2006, pp. 41–48. *MLA International Bibliography/ebsco host.* web 30 Apr 2013.

Sjoblad, Aron. *Metaphorical Coherence.* Lund, Sweden: Lund University Press, 2015.

St. Clair, Robert N. "Language and the Social Construction of Reality." *Language Science,* vol. 4, 1982, pp. 211–236.

St. Clair, Robert N. *Social Metaphor: Essays in Structural Epistemology.* Forthcoming.

Steinitz, Renate. "Adverbial-Syntax." *Studia Grammatica,* 1969, p. 10.

Swinburne, Richard. *The Coherence of Theism.* Oxford: Oxford University Press, 2016.

Tan, K. C., and H. Jeong. "Entanglement as the Symmetric Portion of Correlated Coherence". *Physical Review Letters,* vol. 121, no. 22, 2018, pp. 220401.

Tanskanen, Sanna-Kaisa. *Collaborating towards Coherence: Lexical Cohesion in English Discourse.* Amsterdam: John Benjamin, 2006.

Todd Taylor, ed. *CCCC Bibliography of Composition and Rhetoric 1984–1999. ibiblio.* web 29 Apr 2013.

Toulmin, Stephen. *The Uses of Argument.* Cambridge, England: Cambridge University Press, 1958.

Troup, G. J. *Optical Coherence Theory.* London: Methuen, 1967.

Tuhereze, Elias. "Tribute to Late Prof. Noble Banadda." Makerere University. *https://news.mak.ac.ug/2021/07/tribute-to-late-prof-noble-banadda/.* web July 3, 2021.

Waldron, T. P. *Principles of Language and Mind.* London: Routledge & Kegan Paul, 1985.

Winterowd, Ross. "The Grammar of Coherence." *College English,* vol. 31, May 1970, pp. 828–835.

Witte, Stephen, and Lester Faigley. "Coherence, Cohesion, and Writing Quality." *College Composition and Communication,* vol. 32, 1981, pp. 189–204.

Woodson, Linda. *A Handbook of Modern Rhetorical Terms.* Urbana: NCTE, 1979.

Wyzsocki, Anne, and Dennis Lynch. *The DK Handbook.* Boston: Longman, 2011. Print.

Young, Vershawn Ashanti, Rusty Barrett, Y'Shanda Young-Rivera, and Kim Brian Lovejoy. *Other People's English: Code-Meshing, Code-Switching, and African American Literacy.* New York: Teachers College Press, 2014.

Zaharna, R. S. "Bridging Cultural Differences: American Public Relations Practices & Arab Communication Patterns." *Public Relations Review,* vol. 21, 1995. pp. 241–255.

Index

Agnation 18–20
Alice in Wonderland 14, 60
Aristotle 1, 42

Bamberg, Betty 16, 85, 86
Brannon, Lil see Knoblach and Brannon 60

Carrell, Patricia 14, 61
central cognitive processes 6, 20, 26, 37, 38, 40, 42, 44–48, 55–58, 61, 62, 64, 65, 67–69, 76, 78–80, 82–85, 87, 88, 107
  developmental continuum of 47
  list of 48
  utility of 57
  versatility of 57
central metaphors 6, 26, 59, 60, 62, 67–73, 77, 80, 82, 84, 87
  few in number 67
  guide 46, 67, 89, 101
  isotropism 69
  sensitivity to belief system 46, 67, 68
  touchstone 67
central systems, characteristics of 45, 47
coherence 1–7, 9–11, 13–19, 21, 22, 24, 26, 27, 35–45, 47, 48, 55–64, 70, 73–83, 85–87, 91, 92, 95, 97, 98, 104, 107
  cognitive elements of 6, 35, 57, 60, 62, 76, 78
  definition of 61, 86, 105, 106
  lines of 15, 82
  visual metaphor of 83
cogitation 40
cognition, kinds of 5
cognitive elements of coherence see coherence
cognitive perspective 6, 11, 20, 37–39, 42, 44, 47, 58, 82, 84, 87, 97, 107, 108
cognitive universals 11, 12, 44
contextually salient perspective 19, 20, 59–64, 75, 76, 79, 82, 84, 87, 108
contextually salient elements 26, 35, 75, 76, 79, 82, 83
Corbett, Edward P.J. 5, 73, 81

co-reference 12, 15, 16, 21–23, 27, 58, 82–84, 92–99, 102
  comparative 95, 97, 98
  endophoric 94–96
  exophoric 12, 21, 94–96
  demonstrative 95, 96
  personal 61, 95
culturally salient perspective 6, 62
  paradox 6

de Beaugrande 8, 40, 58
discourse 4, 5, 9, 35, 40, 42, 44, 46, 56, 60, 85, 86, 88

ellipsis 12, 14–16, 21–23, 25, 27, 28, 36, 41, 44, 56, 58, 78–80, 82, 84, 94, 98, 101–107
  form of substitution 98, 107
enation 18–20
epistemological frames 6, 26, 59, 60, 62, 63, 67, 71, 77, 80, 82, 84, 87
Everett, Sakeena 65, 68, 87
explicit-implicit continuum 13, 34, 38, 45, 56, 57, 78, 79, 85, 86
  of linguistic elements 6, 27, 28, 35, 36, 40–44, 56, 57, 60, 62, 78, 82, 83
  of linguistic and cognitive elements 35, 57
  of linguistic, cognitive, and contextually salient elements 35, 79, 82

Fodor, Jerry 9, 45, 68, 69

Gestalt 3, 6, 37, 38, 40, 42–44, 47, 57, 58, 82
  Closure 22, 42, 43, 57, 58, 79, 80, 82, 84
  good continuation 42, 43, 57, 58, 79, 80, 82, 84
  restructuring 42–44, 57, 58, 79, 80, 82, 84
given/new relationship 6, 20, 38, 40–42, 44, 47, 57, 58, 79, 80, 82, 84

Gutwinski, Waldemar 13, 17–22, 26, 27, 36, 76

Halliday and Hasan 8, 13–22, 26, 27, 36, 76, 91–107
Halliday, M.A.K. see Halliday and Hasan 8, 13–22, 26, 27, 36, 76, 91–107
Hasan, Ruquaia see Halliday and Hasan 8, 13–22, 26, 27, 36, 76, 91–107
Hirsch, E.D., Jr. 61
Horace 2, 42

Interpretation 26, 92

Johnson, Mark see Lakoff and Johnson 63, 71

Knoblauch, C.H. see Knoblauch and Brannon 60
Knoblauch and Brannon 60

Lakoff, George 63, 68, 71, 106, 107
Lakoff and Johnson 63, 71
laws of coherence see Hirsch, E.D., Jr. 61
linearity 9–12, 18, 19, 21, 27, 47, 87
linguistic elements of coherence 6, 27, 28, 35, 36, 40, 41, 44, 56, 57, 62, 78
  list of 48
  mandatory explicitness of 36, 56, 78
  names of 27, 28
linguistic perspective 6, 7, 9–13, 16, 18, 21, 24, 27, 34, 37, 41, 42, 56, 75, 78, 82, 84, 92, 98
logical connectors 38
Longinus 2, 3, 42, 81, 83, 89

Markels, Robin B. 13, 21–27, 36
Metaphor 16, 64–69, 71, 72, 77, 83–88
  definition of 64
  cognitive bridging 66
  experiential bridging 66

figures of thought 68
linguistic bridging 65

neoteny 10
nucleus of natural language logic 12, 16, 58, 83, 84, 92
   logical identity 12, 16, 34, 35, 42, 44, 47, 58, 82–84, 92
   symbolic reference 16, 34–36, 47

parallel distributed processing 57, 85
pari passu 11, 34, 47
polysemy 35
   dual nature of 88
pro-forms 16, 28, 35, 36

recurrence (repetition) chains 22
reference 11, 12, 14–16, 18, 19, 21–23, 26, 34–36, 41, 42, 47, 73, 75, 79, 82, 84, 91–94
   anaphora 16, 18–21, 27, 28, 36, 41, 44, 56, 58, 78–80, 82, 84
   cataphora 16, 18–21, 27, 28, 33, 36, 41, 44, 56, 58, 78–80, 82, 84
   exophora 18
   homophora 18, 19
   modal 35, 36, 79
   vs. empirical 12, 35, 36, 46, 63, 68, 76, 79
   paraphora 18, 19
   symbolic function of 12
repetition 14–16, 18–25, 27, 28, 36, 41, 44, 56, 58, 75, 78–80, 82, 84

sociological models 6, 59, 62, 70, 72, 77, 80, 82, 84, 87
   types of 21, 71, 94
speech and writing 8
   differences in 11
sui generis 11
sui species 11, 16
substitution 12, 14–16, 20–23, 28, 94–96, 98–102, 104, 107

symbol 8, 11, 12, 16, 34–36, 40, 47, 61, 70, 71, 73, 92
   functions of 11

teachers 12, 39, 42, 43, 46, 81, 85, 87–89, 105, 106
points of departure for 85
   bottom up and top down processing 86
   culturally salient elements for the good 87
   dual nature of central cognitive processes 88
   linear and non-linear aspects 87
   parts to whole and whole to parts 85, 86
text 1–9, 12–23, 25–27, 35–38, 41–44, 57, 59–62, 68, 76, 78, 79, 81–83, 85–87, 92–95, 97, 100
ties 7–9, 12, 14–16, 20, 21, 93, 94, 100, 107
   basic ties re Halliday and Hasan
   grammatical 11, 18–20, 22, 62, 75, 78, 88, 94, 99
   immediate 8, 27, 47, 93
   lexical 4, 14, 16–18, 20, 22, 94, 99, 107, 108
   remote 27, 93, 94
   of ellipsis 28, 98, 101, 105–107
   of conjunction 107
   of substitution 95, 96, 98–100, 102, 107
   various levels of 75
TG grammar, limit of 25
Toulmin, Stephen E. 41, 73, 74

Warrants 6, 59, 60, 62, 72–76, 78, 80, 82, 84, 87
   field-dependent 74
   field-invariant 73, 74
   register 13, 74, 76, 83, 84, 92, 94, 96
   texture 2, 13, 76, 81
syzygy 81, 88

www.ingramcontent.com/pod-product-compliance
Ingram Content Group UK Ltd.
Pitfield, Milton Keynes, MK11 3LW, UK
UKHW022151230426
12049UKWH00003BA/39